Pregnancy and Childbirth

Books available by the same author

By Appointment Only series:

Arthritis, Rheumatism and Psoriasis
Asthma and Bronchitis
Cancer and Leukaemia
Heart and Blood Circulatory Problems
Migraine and Epilepsy
The Miracle of Life
Multiple Sclerosis
Neck and Back Problems
Realistic Weight Control
Skin Diseases
Stomach and Bowel Disorders
Stress and Nervous Disorders
Traditional Home and Herbal Remedies
Viruses, Allergies and the Immune System
Who's Next?

Nature's Gift Series:

Air – The Breath of Life
Body Energy
Food
Water – Healer or Poison?

Well Woman series:

Menopause
Menstrual and Pre-Menstrual Tension
Pregnancy and Childbirth

The Jan de Vries Healthcare series:

Questions and Answers on Family Health
Life Without Arthritis – the Maori Way

PREGNANCY AND CHILDBIRTH

Jan de Vries

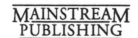

MAINSTREAM
PUBLISHING

EDINBURGH AND LONDON

First published in 1995 by
MAINSTREAM PUBLISHING COMPANY (EDINBURGH) LTD
7 Albany Street
Edinburgh EH1 3UG

ISBN 1 85158 658 X (cloth)
ISBN 1 85158 657 1 (paper)

A catalogue record for this book is available from the British
Library

Typeset in Palatino by Litho Link Ltd, Welshpool, Powys, Wales

Printed and bound in Finland by WSOY

Contents

A baby is God saying that the world should go on

1

Starting a Family

It is 35 years since my wife and I got married, and less than a year later our first child was born. At the time we never thought that this baby would later become a midwife and health visitor. It is hard to put into words the happiness and joy we felt when this baby was born and, when holding my newborn daughter in my arms, it suddenly dawned on me that, as a father, I too was responsible for the well-being of this helpless baby. Three more children were born to us over the years and with all of them we experienced a new happiness and joy that enriched our family.

Not so long ago I returned home from an exhausting series of lectures in the USA. I was very tired and ready to put my feet up, when the telephone rang. I answered it and was surprised to hear my eldest grandchild enquiring how I was. Suddenly it didn't matter how tired I was. What a lovely experience to hear the voice of a young member of the family asking how his grandfather was feeling, and it certainly filled me with joy. I always had a touch of the Peter Pan syndrome and was far from excited at the prospect of becoming a grandfather – until it happened. Indeed, it adds a new dimension to one's life. I remember the day my eldest daughter was born as clearly as I will remember the birth of my first grandchild.

With the greatest pride and joy, as a father to four children and a grandfather to six, I have embarked on writing this book. My eldest daughter, an experienced midwife and herself mother of two children, has given me her support and some practical information for this book. Throughout her study and her career I have been interested in her work. I also decided to talk to one of my favourite patients who is not only a midwife but also a nun. As we had often talked about our work, I was interested to include her views on her work with mothers and babies and asked her to write down some of her experiences. Sister Maria McGuire, who belongs to the Sisters of Wisdom, La Sagesse, has very kindly written down some of her thoughts from the years that she has practised as a midwife, so that we can benefit from her valuable experience. Her balanced view on the subject is very worthwhile, because in her years as a midwife she has been involved in many births and has been closely involved with a great many mothers and babies. Though obviously not a mother herself, she is ideally placed to give us an insight into pregnancy and motherhood from the female point of view, which will complement some of the other views expressed in this book.

Sister Maria writes:

I am deeply interested, and at the same time fascinated, by this wonderfully unique bond of love. Some of the following are my own experiences from working with mostly young pregnant mothers and their 'little ones'. I have used techniques devised by Prof. Terry Dowling, for example:

1. Early bonding as soon as pregnancy was confirmed
2. Asking a two-year-old about who was present at her birth
3. Asking adults, 'Why do you love trees so much?'
4. Using the information and deeper understanding of the deeply intimate relationship of mother and baby to understand problems among young adults, such as rejection
5. Why adoption is such a horrendous decision to make
6. Why miscarriage and still-birth are so traumatic
7. Why post-abortion trauma can be devastating
8. Parenthood and the importance of a family

For the sake of brevity I will use one example for each of the above categories, and to preserve confidentiality I will use fictitious names.

1. Early Bonding

Judith was a young native African girl. She was unmarried and about five months pregnant. She was looking forward to the birth of her baby very much, so we discussed various ways of facilitating and deepening her bonding. This she eagerly took to. I encouraged her to talk to the little one about everything she would normally chat about, saying, 'It's a lovely day' and 'I love you very much', etc.

I also encouraged her to caress the baby by gently stroking and massaging her fairly large tummy and then allowing her hand to rest on her tummy, so that the little one could snuggle into her hand. Also, doing this simple exercise in the comfort of a nice relaxing bath is very soothing to both mother and child.

Judith had a healthy baby boy. He was a very contented baby and his birth was quick and uncomplicated. Judith had a very short term of labour. She was delighted with her baby, was in good health and very happy.

With my own input in working in pregnancy care, every child has known my voice, but obviously their mum's voice was the favourite. Where possible I have included the fathers, but sadly only a very small number stayed by the side of their girlfriend.

2. Who was at your birth?

While on a home visit to assess and observe mother and daughter, the subject of Jane's birth was introduced by her mother. I felt this was a good opportunity to ask two-year-old Jane some questions. She was an intelligent and very articulate child, so I asked, 'Jane, who was with you when you were born?' Jane, without hesitation, replied, 'My Gran.' Then her mother said, 'No Jane, that was my gran, your great-grandmother.' Well, two-year-old Jane became very annoyed and was adamant, 'No, she is my gran.' Mum soothed her and said, 'Okay Jane, she is your gran.' I asked Jane if there was anyone else there and shyly she looked at her mother and said, 'My mum.'

3. I love to ask people 'Why do we love trees so much?'

Personally, I feel delighted to be among trees. They are so strong, yet gentle; they make me feel secure and protected. I love to stand gazing at the sky through the branches, especially if the tree is a big sturdy oak. I know I was loved and cherished from conception. My two older brothers wanted a baby sister, so they prayed to God for me. There is a theory that babies can actually see before birth, and another about what it is they actually see *first*. In my personal experience, and perhaps in many other people's, I am sure it was a tree. That is one reason why so many beautiful things have been written about trees.

9

4. Relationship in the womb between mother and baby to understand problems which people express and manifest in later life

I have worked with approximately 400 young women during their pregnancies. Many were in residential care due to concealed pregnancies where the baby was to go for adoption or difficult family situations which made it necessary for the girls to go into residential care during the remainder of their pregnancy. For the majority, the problems eventually evaporated and their families gave their support in varying degrees.

I found that those girls who had the most problems had themselves been rejected by one or both parents. Their ability to trust people was sadly shattered. When love and care was given, this was tested, usually by the girl being more demanding and causing more problems. Those who tested the carers without being rejected (as they expected to be) actually began to trust them. However, there were a number of girls who did not know what ordinary family life was, as they had been in care since infancy and, although they learned good parenting skills, they needed ongoing affirmation and support to help them to rear their own children.

I could not resolve their situation, or rather their experience of life, but I could assist them to look at the various reasons why they experienced parental rejection. This was done by looking at the lifestyles of their own parents prior to marriage, and studying their own family network and history. Often spouses work out marital problems through 'scapegoating' their children. Explaining this can give young girls an informed knowledge of what had been happening to them and raise their confidence, self-esteem and understanding.

Girls who had experienced the trauma of rejection by their mother or father, but especially by their mother, would seek love and affection from any man who appeared to offer this. However, the majority of these relationships ended in tragedy and violence. The girl would be left alone and pregnant. She would consequently seek love for herself in her baby.

5. Adoption

I have seen about sixty girls agonise over whether or not to choose adoption for their child. It is not a decision lightly made. A great deal of counselling is given to assist the girl in making the best decision for her baby. This is because she is caring for her little one and wants only the very best family, where this child will be loved, wanted and given a good start in life.

Carol and Philip were two students, each with their future mapped out. Although Carol was pregnant, they decided that they were too young to take on the responsibility of a child, so they both wanted adoption. Their attitude to the baby, however, was saying, 'We really want this child.' This baby was loved in the womb by both his mum and dad, but they both remained adamant that adoption was the only choice as they both planned to go to university.

Sadly, prior to the baby's birth, the young father became very ill. He was suffering from leukaemia and he was dying. Eventually Carol took her baby son out of foster care (incidentally, no one knew of this baby's existence in either family) and went to see Philip in hospital. Philip was delighted to see his son and managed to smile. He was so weak that he was no longer able to talk. Carol was a very courageous girl and had great inner strength. She took her son to meet both families – what a reunion this was. Tears of delight were shed and families rallied round. Sadly, Philip did not survive his illness, but his mother, though grief-stricken, rejoiced in her grandson. God's ways are not our ways.

6. Miscarriage and still-birth

Society in Britain expects parents, especially mothers, to wash their faces, put on fresh make-up and carry on as normal when tragedies such as miscarriage occur. Our society cannot cope with this kind of grief, so people's advice is, 'Just forget it ever happened – you can always have another baby.' Another baby – yes. This little one – no! This one is irreplaceable and parents know this. Mothers need to share their deep hurt and work through their grief. Otherwise, if left in isolation, depression can set in, or they begin to think that what they are feeling is abnormal and that they are really going mad. This child was living with them and was a person, loved and wanted, no matter how little he or she was.

A few mothers I knew miscarried around the same time, so they welcomed the opportunity to come together to share their grief. They were angry at the insensitive way they and their miscarried children were treated by the medical profession. Even their husbands refused to discuss the babies. Fathers feel very deeply for their little ones too, but often cannot bring themselves to talk about how they feel. I think this is because society demands that men be strong – they cannot afford to cry, and this is really what would do them a power of good. In the group we talked together, we cried together; all feelings were freely expressed.

7. Abortion

I feel very deeply for mothers subjected to this devastating trauma. It is a known fact that at approximately 12 weeks' gestation the mother usually suffers from depression, and it is precisely at this stage that she has to make an unenviable decision. No one else can share such a horrendous decision – only the mother. Studies have shown that many women suffer at some time in their lives from post-abortion trauma. This devastates that person and can ruin her life utterly and entirely if she is not given the right help and compassion.

The psychological and physical effects can be devastating. Yes, many women receive counselling and psychological assessment prior to abortion, but it is important who is there that they receive sympathetic care afterwards. Some women who have suffered from the aftermath of abortion feel the void left by someone who has lived with them for a short time. Their grief is sometimes harrowing; guilt weighs heavily, and who, they wonder, could forgive them. God is all compassion and love, slow to anger and rich in mercy. He alone knows the depths of the suffering of these mothers – He forgives. Their child, who is with God, also forgives, and the mother has to come to accept forgiveness and to forgive herself.

8. Parenthood

The roles of mothers and fathers are of prime importance to their children. Children are the fruit of the love each has for the other, and children thrive, grow and learn from this. The dignity and rights of the family are the roots of any country. Sadly, many countries throughout the world have eroded the status of parents making it meaningless, and outdated. Career hunting and social status have become the rule for many. However, there is much hope to be gained from seeing parents actively taking on their roles in a responsible manner, seriously and in love.

Fathers are often left out in the cold during pregnancy. Their bonding and relationship with their child is also crucial, and they must work together with their wives to achieve this. This intimate bond of union is so beautiful, but needs to be communicated, protected and nurtured.

The thoughts of Sister Maria are reflected in the Ten Child Care Commandments in the book *The Needs of Children* by Dr Mia Pringle:

1. Give loving care
2. Give time and talk to your child
3. Encourage play
4. Praise effort
5. Give responsibility
6. Remember your child is unique
7. Let your disapproval of your child's temperament be positive
8. Don't make him/her feel pushed aside
9. Never threaten to stop loving
10. Don't expect gratitude – your child did not ask to be born

'When one cannot feel safe in the mother's bosom, there is no place left to feel safe.' I was reminded of this quotation when I read the book *The Magical Child* written by Joseph Shilton Pierce. This book was given to me by the owner of a healthfood store who attended one of my lectures with her child. She told me that she had been very impressed with this book and I too have read it with great pleasure. Certainly nothing can equal or replace the safety of a mother's bosom, and growing up in the knowledge that our mother is there when we are in need of advice, develops a secure bond. Age does not come into it – a mother will always hold that position in the life of her child. This bond or rapport between a mother and her child depends on the development of their relationship over the years and generally a mother will intuitively know how to deal with her child's insecurities.

Exceptions or excesses are possible if this relationship is handled incorrectly and as a result I have seen many instances of the so-called 'Oedipus complex'. This is a situation where the child is very attached to the parent of the opposite sex and is frequently hostile towards the other parent. Very often such a relationship remains unresolved even in adulthood. In *The Magical Child* the writer claims that such feelings are usually based on a monstrous misunderstanding which remains significant in the future relationship of the child towards others.

Back in the 1940s, two researchers, Bernard and Sontag, found that the infant *in utero* immediately responded with body movement to sounds from its mother and to sounds in her immediate environment. In 1970, researchers Brody and Axelwort stated

13

categorically that there were no random movements in the newborn or uterine infant. Every movement, they insisted, has meaning, purpose and design. Within minutes of birth the newborn baby begins almost continuous movements of its limbs, body and head.

I once heard an interesting story about a woman whose husband practised medicine. They worked in Uganda many years ago, and when the local mothers brought their infants to see the doctor they had to wait patiently in line for hours. The women carried these tiny infants in a sling next to their bare breast and no diapers or nappies were used. Yet, it seemed that none of the infants was soiled when it was their time to be examined by the doctor. The doctor's wife wondered how these women could manage to keep their infants so clean. The women explained that they just temporarily left the queue and disappeared into the bushes, but this still left the doctor's wife wondering how they knew when it was time for the infant to relieve itself. She was then told that a mother knew instinctively when her infant was going to urinate or defecate. The psychologist Karl Jung said that the child lives in the unconscious of the parent and, when we look at the above, it seems that Jung was correct in this theory. A conscious parent encompasses the psychological state of the child – the intuition is highly tuned.

It was noted by the researcher Blurton Jones that breast-fed infants cry more than bottle-fed infants, but only during the first year of their lives. Thereafter, the breast-fed infants cry far less than those who are bottle-fed. This shows that breast-feeding establishes a bond during the first year of life.

It is important that the parents-to-be are aware of these facts when they decide to start a family and consider the role of both partners in this process. She conceives because she wants to create life, as her intent drives her. Also, when it is her first pregnancy, the fact that she has been found to be fertile and that she will soon give birth is a source of strength to her and provides a positive energy flow. But the man too has to provide a vital and calming influence. It is important that there is a bond, and the strength and support of a husband or mate is almost essential for an anxiety-free pregnancy and motherhood. The strength of the father must feed into the mother, and through her into the new life. This support and understanding between the partners will be the foundation of a happy family.

Assuming the pregnancy is planned, what is the process when a couple decides to start a family? Much talk takes place and no doubt the financial aspects of the situation are weighed up. Both partners have their own views on the future and will try to see themselves in their new role. In other words, they prepare themselves for the future, as they have planned it. Even if the pregnancy is unplanned, the partners still have nine months to prepare themselves before the birth. The sequence of events each partner lives through in the case of an unplanned pregnancy is significant in the development of their attitude towards the responsibility for a new life and their readiness to make sacrifices for the sake of an infant they may not yet have come to love.

As a father of four I have found this one of the most intriguing emotions one faces in life. Something profound happens the moment you learn that you are going to be a parent, and whether or not it is the first time makes little or no difference. This is not surprising if one considers the development during the early stages of an embryo. Suppose that the embryo is approximately six weeks old by the time the pregnancy is suspected or confirmed. By that time the embryo already has eyes and is about 13 mm long. This is when the wonder of nature becomes apparent, because conception takes place in darkness, in the womb of the mother.

Life starts with one very small egg cell and a sperm cell fifty thousand times smaller than the egg cell. I find it fascinating that millions of sperm cells reach the egg, but only one is able to penetrate. It takes four weeks for the egg cell to change to an embryo, and by that time it has grown to ten thousand times its original size. During that time this embryo already has its own heart. A newly born baby girl already has 500,000 egg cells of her own. When this girl has reached the age of thirteen there are only 10,000 egg cells left, and from this age onwards one of the ripe cells travels from the ovaries each month, which is called ovulation. This usually takes place between the times of menstruation; fourteen days after menstruation an egg begins a journey which ends fourteen days after the next menstruation. This is what is thought to be the most fertile period.

Thinking about a family and its preparation, the adult womb prepares itself every month for pregnancy. Between 45 million and 700 million sperm cells are released during intercourse and there is a race to see which one will fertilise the egg cell. Sometimes the sperm cells live for two days or even a little longer. At the moment of fertilisation the colour of the hair, the eyes and the skin are determined, and within half an hour of fertilisation there will already be a division of cells. The sex is determined by the sperm cell. The pregnancy can be determined three weeks after fertilisation. After thirty days every organ begins to grow and after the twenty-fifth day the heart of the foetus starts to beat. The embryo feeds from the mother via the placenta. After 12 weeks the foetus is about 2.5 cm long and weighs about 20 g. Nine weeks after fertilisation the foetus has its own unique fingerprints. And so the process goes on.

In the second month the foetus already has eyes, nose, ears, a mouth and a tongue. In this stage the brain and bone marrow grow faster than any of the other organs so that the embryo, in comparison with the rest of the body, has quite a big head. Only six weeks after fertilisation teeth begin to appear. In the third month the embryo is beginning to look more human and towards the end of the month the foetus can move, swallow, stretch its toes, make a fist, and it can also move its head. When the mother feels that there is a new life inside her, it is a wonderful experience.

After these first three months the baby has developed considerably and, although it is no longer than 7.5 cm, it is already recognisably human. All the organs are formed, the muscles and nerves are functioning and even the baby's reflexes are good. The heart pumps 25 litres of blood through the body daily.

During the fourth month the foetus grows to about 12 cm and its weight will be around 100 g. It can live quite easily in the womb, being nourished by the placenta or afterbirth. Much research on the placenta has been done, and if the mother were to develop any problems at this stage of her pregnancy, this could be detected in the placenta, if it were checked after the baby was born.

I remember the birth of my first child took place at home and my friend and colleague who assisted at the birth was very interested to see the afterbirth, which is about 20 to 36 cm in size. My wife had had considerable problems with her blood pressure during pregnancy and from the afterbirth we could see exactly what had happened as it not only showed her circulatory patterns but also graphically revealed how the blood pressure of the foetus had changed during the pregnancy.

At the beginning of the fifth month the baby is about 30 cm long and 500 g in weight. Now the mother can easily feel the baby's movement; the bones and nails are hardening and the muscles are developing and getting stronger. In the sixth month hair growth and an increase of body fat takes place. It is now possible for the baby to breathe outside the womb.

During the next three months the baby develops steadily and becomes more independent. In the seventh month it gains, on average, another two pounds, while during the last six weeks or so it will possibly gain another four pounds. If all is well, the weight of the baby will grow steadily.

In the last weeks before birth, growth continues until the baby fills the womb and its movements are restricted due to lack of space. The birth of the baby is calculated to be approximately 280 days from the first day of the last menstruation. As a generalisation, this is the nearest estimate doctors can give because the menstruation or the fertile period may have been slightly irregular.

What exactly happens during the birth process is still a mystery. There are theories that suggest there are mechanical stimulations, or that at the end of the pregnancy the uterus becomes very sensitive, or that the head of the unborn baby begins to cause pressure on the uterus. Or, perhaps, there may be reflexes in the bowels which induce labour. Another theory claims that there is a change in the hormone, and it is believed that giving one or more injections of oxytocin causes the hypophysis, or pituitary gland in the brain, to secrete a hormone which speeds up the birth of the baby. I must say, however, that I am totally against this. The more natural way in which we handle a pregnancy and a birth, the better, and as with all hormone preparations, one should treat them very carefully as we do not always know what the outcome may be. The prevalent theory is that the uterus contracts and that there are chemical changes for both mother and child and certain ingredients are produced by the body to start the birth process spontaneously. Sometimes labour begins too early or too late and I have seen this occur with my own children: one of them was early, while another was late. Luckily, there was never any sign of a miscarriage, although at one point, when my wife joined me on an overseas flight when she was about 20 weeks into her pregnancy, she suffered fairly heavy bleeding. Fortunately, a miscarriage was avoided and the foetus was unaffected.

The placenta grows quickly with the foetus and must function correctly if the baby is to develop healthily. The uterus should be in good condition so that there is a regular blood supply – essential for the development of the placenta and the growing foetus. Wounds or small mishaps will rarely affect the pregnancy, but the thalidomide situation in the early sixties taught us that the foetus can be damaged by external influences. This harsh lesson revealed how important it is to check what kind of remedies or medicines the mother takes, or what kind of treatment is used, as chemicals and X-rays can have a detrimental effect on the foetus. Therefore, herbal and homoeopathic remedies, which are gentle and safe, are very much preferred to most other medications.

I wish I was able to describe the feelings of elation and joy that pervade when the baby arrives. It is such a wonderful event and I am so pleased that, with all four of our children, I was able to be present at the birth. It is also a very humbling experience. Every day on this earth, new life is created and with this new creation comes fresh hope and promise for the future. Only the Creator of mankind knows how it really works.

'Before I formed you in the womb I knew you and before you come out of the womb I sanctified you'

Jeremiah Ch. 1: v. 5

Looking at a newborn baby, we wonder if such a little creature can feel emotions, or if it has thoughts, because everything it does seems to be done intuitively. We watch it while it is asleep and see that it enjoys a restful and peaceful sleep. We wonder if the baby dreams. If it cries, does it know that it is because of hunger, or because of discomfort? It knows that to suck its thumb provides comfort. We look in wonder and amazement at its little mannerisms and are fascinated by the rapid stages of development. The little newcomer intuitively looks to its mother to be fed and a pattern of activity quickly develops. Reflexes are obvious from movements such as the baby's clenching and unclenching its hands, moving its arms about in instinctive punching and stretching movements, and kicking its legs. Even at birth their strength is quite amazing, especially in their legs. When you lift a baby so that his or her feet are on your thighs, you soon realise how strong the leg muscles are because the baby will instinctively kick out, as if trying to take its weight on its own feet. The same with their little fists: if you let a baby put its fist around your little finger you will feel its strength when it grips that finger.

The routine reflex of the baby is intuitively to look for food. The baby can smell and taste and, although its brain is a quarter of the size of an adult's, it is surprising to see how well the baby's reflexes function. Research has shown that a newborn child can focus on an object and follow movements. After six to eight weeks the baby can tell whether things are close to hand or further away. With our babies, I was always intrigued by the perpetual movements of their hands and the perfectly formed miniature details, such as the fingernails. I doubt if we will ever know what a little baby thinks or senses. It is quite something to see a baby of four to six weeks smiling, especially when it sees its own mother.

Their activity and their different interests and rate of development is, and always will be, a mystery to me. Take my two youngest grandchildren: one was born totally bald, while the other had such an abundant mop of hair that it was remarked on by

18

everyone. It is a mystery how every newborn child has common reflexes and, yet, is so different. Certainly, we know that infants can hear, smell, taste, see, and drink, but I was amazed to see one of my children, when only twelve hours old, literally clinging to her mother. I wonder what emotional changes take place in a mother during pregnancy, and if she is aware of them. I appreciate that this must be dependent on how the mother experiences and enjoys her pregnancy. Social acceptance of her pregnancy is also important, for example, is she and her pregnancy accepted by those people around her? Are those people, together with the mother-to-be, looking forward to this happy event? Although pregnancy is a totally natural, biological process, sometimes emotional upsets can affect the mother to an extent which may affect the baby. When awaiting the arrival of a first baby, the role of the father is of particular importance.

Not so long ago I treated a young woman whose happiness in her pregnancy was overshadowed by fear. Her mother had told her so many frightful things about childbirth that she had become extremely nervous at the very thought of her own delivery. It took a lot of reasoning and discussion before she accepted that it is a completely natural event which leaves every woman with memories that are uniquely hers. Sometimes I have had to prescribe remedies for young pregnant women to help them to balance their emotional feelings and apprehensions about the birth because they cannot look beyond the fact that there is a lot of pain involved.

Pregnancy can also bring out feelings of guilt. For whatever reason they arise, whether founded or not, if the expectant mother develops these feelings, the condition of both mother and baby will be affected. As a father-to-be, with every child my wife was expecting, I had to cope with a fear or concern, which I never dared share with my wife, that the child would be healthy. Perhaps I was prone to such fears because I have practised medicine for so long and have seen so many things which can go wrong. However, I have always tried to hide these feelings from my wife, and later from my daughters. It is worse if the mother-to-be has these worries because this can add to the strain. Having said that, I am sure that most women also experience these fears, which are quite natural, but manage to keep them under control.

Nine months can be a very long time and sometimes I have great difficulty in convincing the expectant mother that pregnancy and childbirth is a natural process, which will progress according to nature's ways. It is true that the hormonal changes in the expectant mother are mostly positive. Endorphins and encephalins are

19

released spontaneously and many previously rheumatic or arthritic women have reported a pregnancy totally free of those symptoms. This was perhaps due to the beneficial impact of these naturally released hormonal ingredients. In most cases, pregnancy and the process of birth is a cleansing process for women with medical conditions.

When a woman is expecting her second or third child, she will have to consider how to deal with her other children. The mother may be worried whether the newborn baby will be accepted or will cause jealousy among the other children. It is not uncommon for similar feelings to be experienced by a new father. The relationship between the mother-to-be and the other members of the family must be a mutually supportive one.

I have often spoken with fathers who felt rejected by their wives because too many women are ill-informed and believe that sex during pregnancy is wrong. It could be that these misunderstandings are fostered because the mother-to-be feels disinclined towards sex during her pregnancy, but unless there is a medical condition indicating that it would be safer for either mother or baby if no sex took place, having sex at this time is perfectly safe. Any disinclination might be temporary, due to a hormonal change, but nature definitely does not dictate that sexual relationships should cease. Everything can be completely normal – unless the woman has previously displayed a tendency to miscarry or has suffered bleedings. In those cases it is important to remember that fourteen weeks after conception the foetus will be well established and therefore only during the first three months should special care be taken. I would suggest, if there are any such problems, that the mother-to-be speaks to her own doctor or goes to a midwife for advice. In some cases a marriage has been badly affected by these misunderstandings. After the birth of the baby it is sensible not to re-start the usual sexual relationship for the first six weeks, after which everything should be back to normal.

The first month after such a happy occasion can be one of great contentment as mother and baby become used to each other; but always remember to include the father and the other children in the family in this bond. Together, they can give the newcomer a caring and loving start in the world. I remember how proud I was with every child we had and how proud I have been at the birth of each of my grandchildren.

A newborn baby – helpless and small as it is – gives parents and other children feelings of love, tenderness and great pride. It is important that babies are fed correctly, have sufficient sleep and all the loving care possible. New mothers will soon learn what to do when their baby cries. There is no reason to be upset about this, because it is perfectly natural and happens to all babies; usually a baby crying is no more than a signal, indicating hunger, a wet nappy, wind, and so on.

Practical considerations for a baby's comfort include using the correct weight and thickness of clothing, and maintaining the right temperature and atmosphere. Avoid draughts so that it is less likely for the baby to catch a cold, and make sure that the baby is not subjected to drastic temperature changes. Use clean, lukewarm water to wash a baby's head and face, but soap is not always necessary and quite often the baby's skin is too sensitive. If you prefer to use soap, use only a mild baby-soap, and make sure that the residue is well rinsed off with clean water. If the baby has diarrhoea, more than usual care should be taken not to further irritate the skin with unsuitable soap products. There are some excellent mild cleansing-lotions, specifically designed for sensitive baby skin, which cleanse and soothe. Remember that too much washing may destroy the natural oils in the skin tissue. Tender areas such as the ears, mouth and nose, should be cleaned very gently and lotions, creams and ointments are often only needed if the skin is damaged.

The choice of nappies is much better nowadays, and disposable nappies are indeed a great discovery. I still vividly remember trying to be helpful and changing the nappy for one of my daughters. In my inexperience I pricked our daughter with the safety-pin. At least this risk is now non-existent with modern disposable nappies.

A baby requires around five or six feeds every 24 hours. A feed should not normally take longer than half an hour, nor should the time taken for bathing.

The ideal birth-weight for a boy should be around 4–5 kg and for a girl from 3½ to 4½ kg. At the clinic you will be told what the expected weight gain of your baby should be and a close eye will be kept on this.

Constipation is usually the result of incorrect feeding, and diarrhoea in a baby should be treated very quickly, because persistent diarrhoea carries the risk of dehydration. A young baby's motion should be of a yellowish colour. When the motion turns a greenish shade, it can indicate an infection, while small dark-green motions can be a sign of insufficient feeding.

As an osteopath I would stress that the baby's mattress should be firm. This is not only important for the development of the baby's vertebrae, but also to avoid the risk of suffocation.

Although it is sometimes a healthy sign if the baby cries, constant crying can indicate certain problems. With one of my children, who cried constantly for six weeks, we were on our last legs, until we found that for some inexplicable reason breast-feeding was not sufficient and she needed supplementary feeding. This is often the reason why I sympathise with young mothers when they come to see me and ask why their babies are crying so much, even though every effort has been taken to keep the baby happy and content. An adult cries because of pain or sadness, but to a baby, crying is the only way it is able to communicate its feelings. It is a good sign when the baby cries immediately after the birth. This way the doctor or midwife can check if the breathing, lungs and voice are all right. After a few weeks, a baby starts to produce real tears and sometimes it cries to attract the mother's attention. From the very beginning, a baby associates its mother with food, warmth and safety. When the baby breathes deeply and starts to cry, the mother will usually have a fair idea why her baby is crying. Often, in its haste to satisfy its hunger, the baby will gulp too much air when feeding, and will need help to rid itself of the wind which causes flatulence. Usually a baby is crying because it either feels unhappy, uncomfortable or perhaps wants to communicate that it feels lonely.

Some time ago I had a patient who came to me completely frustrated and worn out because she claimed that her baby had been crying for three months. Eventually, it was discovered what was wrong: the baby was allergic to something in the atmosphere of its bedroom. It transpired that the starch in the new curtains in the room gave off a distinct vapour. This conclusion was reached by a process of elimination – when the baby was put to sleep elsewhere, it slept well. After the curtains had been washed, ridding them of the starch, the baby slept happily in its bedroom. Sometimes, therefore, situations that appear to be disastrous, can be overcome by minor adjustments, because all too often small details are overlooked.

I have already mentioned that parental stress can be caused by a frequently crying baby, but how do parents cope with a hyperactive child? One of my grandchildren is the most active and energetic child I have ever come across. She simply does not want to go to sleep, and she is a very light sleeper so that even the slightest sound is enough to wake her. Once awake, it is hard to coax her to go back to sleep because she wants company and wants to talk. Fortunately, her mother is understanding and although it is tiring for her, she will attend to the child and try to settle her again. It is really quite remarkable to see how quickly children pick up the vibrations and emotions from the mother and interpret these as positive or negative.

Sometimes the crying of a baby is reassuring. Many a new mother has crept up to the cradle or cot to see if all is well. However, never is the sound of your baby's cry more welcome than at the birth.

The birth process takes place in three stages, the first of which is when the cervix begins to dilate. The pains and contractions become stronger during the second stage, and the baby presses more and begins to force its way into the birth canal. If the blood circulation is not interrupted and the baby receives the right amount of oxygen, the baby then slowly makes its way out through the birth canal. When the head has reached the widest part of the vagina, it usually progresses quickly from there on. Recent research indicates that the child is not totally inactive during the actual birth process. Immediately the baby has left the mother's body, the air passages must be cleared of all mucus and fluid to enable the baby to breathe on its own. During this special moment the first breath of life floods into the lungs and, after this first gulp of air, surely the most welcome sound to a mother must be to hear her baby cry.

2

Food Management

My wife and I were most concerned because one of our daughters cried day and night. This went on for about six weeks before we finally discovered that, for some inexplicable reason, she was not getting sufficient nourishment from her food. The poor little thing did not actually have the very best start in life. First of all, drugs were needed to assist her entry into the world. Next, because both my wife and I believe in breast-feeding, we persevered with this without realising that this baby was not receiving enough nutrition from the milk. We did not realise this until it became obvious that this little girl was not gaining sufficient weight. When the problem was identified and remedied, we were delighted to see that, fortunately, she showed no detrimental signs as a result of her early hunger pangs, and she grew into a strong and healthy child.

The first and most important form of food is breast-milk. I have admired my wife when I have seen how difficult this was for her. I have seen her persevere even when her nipples were raw; she would insist on feeding her baby herself. During the first month, in particular, there may be some problems while mother and baby get to know each other. At times I have been utterly amazed at the strength of this bond, this natural drive in a mother. Even when my wife was really quite ill, the production of milk still continued. The quality of the milk was not affected, and the baby thrived, despite the fact that my wife went through a period of illness and prolonged tiredness. I still feel that one of the most wonderful gifts of nature is that most mothers, no matter what the circumstances, are able, if they wish, to feed their own child. Because of this miracle of nature I am sad when I see female patients who are not prepared to give their baby the best possible start in life. There are women who have some strange ideas about breast-feeding and some who actually have an aversion to it. It fills me with great joy when I visit countries in the Third World and see how mothers feed their babies. Most children who are breast-fed reap the benefits in later life.

I have been asked so often how I can work such long hours and still be fit and energetic. Deep down in my heart I thank my mother for my stamina. In her day, my mother was something of a social outcast as it was considered excessive to breast-feed your baby beyond a certain age. However, my mother has told me that I was breast-fed for an unusually long time, because there was very little food about and, therefore, little option. I am quite sure, even though it was rarely appreciated in those days, that her wisdom, when food was scarce, gave me the best possible start in life. I have worked in countries where infectious diseases are rife, and yet I have never been affected by them; and I am sure that my mother's fortitude has enriched my life with a great immune system.

Only too often mothers ask my help for children with unidentified skin diseases or asthma problems, and I discover that as a baby the child was bottle-fed. The important factor here is that cow's milk contains nine times more protein than mother's milk and the baby, being bombarded with all this protein, cannot cope with it and often develops infantile eczema, or other asthmatic conditions. Added to this, cow's milk produces excessive mucus which causes babies to become congested – one of the worst conditions that can affect a baby. After all, many elderly people die from congestion and, by not giving the baby the best possible start, mothers could unintentionally inflict this condition on their child; a condition that could stay with them for the rest of their lives.

Breast-feeding is important, and the ability of a mother to do so successfully, is greatly dependent on the mother's food management during her pregnancy. Complications are possible, perhaps because of a mother's allergy to certain foods. Also, some knowledge of food-combining is helpful. An expectant mother's diet should contain plenty of fruit, vegetables and nuts, which have all the nutrients that are beneficial to her during pregnancy, and for the development of a healthy child. I have frequently come across health conditions in babies which are indirectly linked to the mother continuing to drink alcohol or to smoke during pregnancy. Some mothers even continue taking drugs while pregnant and I have been horrified listening to some of the stories my daughter, who is a midwife, has had to tell. She has had to deliver children whose fathers and mothers were drug-addicts. These children's health is affected both physically and mentally, and other midwives have asked me to stress the importance of an expectant mother's food management.

The first question a mother usually asks after she is delivered of her baby is, if everything is all right. However, the very best protection the parents can give their future children is their own good health, even before pregnancy begins. As it takes two to make a baby, the health of both parents is important. The man's sperm is as pertinent to the baby's health as the woman's eggs and lifestyle. Smoking, drinking, drug abuse or pollution, are factors that can influence the health of the baby. Throughout life, thousands of cells are continuously dying off and a good diet is vital in the manufacture of healthy cells to replace the old cells. Fresh food is very important in this process.

Any food that is heated, tinned and mixed with white sugar loses its value. Potatoes, on the other hand, are of great value for a pregnant mother as they contain ingredients that are like building-blocks for the baby's health. If the mother-to-be can eat fruit and vegetables grown under responsible conditions, the nutrients will improve the health of both mother and child. The same principle applies to grains. If they are grown without the use of artificial fertilisers and pesticides, their nutritional value is so much higher. Sugary products, sweets, biscuits, cakes, fizzy drinks, and foods that contain additives have no place in a wholesome diet. I often wonder how people kept their food before we discovered preservatives. Salting or pickling may not have been to everyone's taste, but certainly no additives were used, as is the case today. Our palates have become quite used to the taste of preservatives, colourings, emulsifiers, sweeteners, antioxidants, and so on, but that does not mean that additives are harmless. I must emphasise that they are no good to newborn babies.

Sugar must also be one of the worst enemies to a pregnant woman. Not only because of the inevitable weight problems, but because sugar affects the calcium content in the body from the moment it is ingested. Since I consciously decided to cut sugar from my diet, I have been amazed to discover how many food products contain artificial sweeteners. Most of the sugars we eat are hidden in foods where we do not expect to find any sweeteners. Manufacturers add sugar to a great many types of food and it would be frightening to add up our total intake of these hidden sugars. Since I have cut out sugar, I have lost a considerable amount of weight without dieting, and I feel very much better for it.

When you go shopping, check the labels. Cut down on snacks like sweets and fizzy drinks between meals, and you will feel the benefit. Refined sugars do very little for your energy levels, apart from giving them a short-lived boost. Never give a baby a dummy dipped in a sweetened drink, because the baby's palate will very soon get used to something sweet as a pacifier, and it will become more difficult to cut this out in later life. Furthermore, think of the harm this does to a toddler's teeth.

Cereals and bread play an important part in a well-managed food pattern. Always ask for wholemeal flour, muesli and wholemeal biscuits. A baby developing in the mother's womb thrives on regular nourishment, and when a woman is pregnant, long gaps without food will only make her feel sick.

Smoking should definitely be stopped during pregnancy and, better still, before the pregnancy starts. If one feels that it cannot be achieved without help try acupuncture treatment which has helped a lot of people. In a fact sheet that was passed on to me by a patient, it was explained that people smoke for a number of reasons. Some are unhappy and think that it may cheer them up. Other people are bored and think, 'When life is a drag . . . have a fag.' Some are curious, or feel they want to fit in with the crowd they mix with, and therefore start to smoke. Nicotine is a drug and one is much wiser never to even start smoking.

I read an interesting article in the *Daily Telegraph* on 14 April 1992, written by Christine Doyle, which gave dietary guidelines for pregnant women. It stated that excess alcohol or occasional binge drinking can cause defects in the unborn child. And it suggested a limit of three or four cups of coffee a day for pregnant women, while people with blood pressure problems should not drink coffee at all. Fish is generally believed to improve one's IQ, although there is no scientific evidence for this. However, oily fish, such as mackerel, provide a good source of vitamin A. Green or jacket potatoes are not recommended because of a possible link with spina bifida, and pregnant women should eat their potatoes peeled and thoroughly cooked.

The article also contained some good advice for cheese-eaters. There are some very extreme thoughts about cheese but, generally, avoid ripened, soft cheeses, such as Brie and Camembert, blue-veined cheeses, such as Stilton, Shropshire and Roquefort, and goat and sheep cheeses. All hard, Cheddar-style cheeses, soft process-spreads and cream-cheeses are fine. There is some confusion on the subject of yoghurt and yoghurt-based dips and sauces, but the golden rule is to avoid unpasteurised milk, whether it be from a cow, a sheep or a goat, unless it has been boiled. Again, avoid pâté unless this is specifically marked as being pasteurised. Salmonella food poisoning has been linked with eggs and with undercooked poultry. Shellfish should also be avoided because of the increased risk of salmonella and other forms of food poisoning. Although it is thought that this condition will not directly affect the foetus, the vomiting and sickness are distressing during pregnancy. Eating undercooked meat would present a 1:50,000 chance that the baby would contact toxoplasmosis, an infection that can lead to severe learning difficulties and blindness, and therefore it makes sense not to eat raw or undercooked meat. Also, be careful with pre-cooked, chilled meals, some of which are known to cause lysteria. Liver is not recommended during pregnancy because of the increased risk of abnormalities as a result of the very high levels of vitamin A. For the same reason megadoses of any vitamin are not advisable during pregnancy. Eat plenty of green vegetables, fortified breakfast cereals and foods with a high content of Folic Acid. Vegetarians should be especially careful with their diet and supplements of B12 may be necessary.

In my opinion, this article contained some very sensible dietary advice indeed. The body is 80 per cent alkaline and 20 per cent acid. Most people have a high acid-level and so, particularly during pregnancy, alkaline-rich foods are important, such as fresh fruits, vegetables, seeds, nuts and so on. It should not be forgotten that over-nutrition is as big a problem to one's health as malnutrition.

If the pregnant woman suffers from allergic problems she should give some serious thought to food-combining. More detailed information on this subject can be found in my book *Nature's Gift of Food*. Here, I will only concern myself with how the digestion can be made easier and more efficient, always remembering that the simpler the meal, the better one feels.

Foods that contain a high percentage of proteins require an acid-digestive medium. Therefore, the following rules on food-combining should be understood:

1. Avoid eating carbohydrates with acid fruits, and also avoid the combination of concentrated proteins with concentrated carbohydrates.
2. Do not consume two concentrated proteins at the same meal. Since concentrated protein is more difficult to digest than other food elements, concentrated proteins of a different character and composition, such as nuts and cheese, should not be combined.
3. Do not consume fats in the same meal as protein, because our need for concentrated fats is small and most protein foods already contain a good deal of fats. Fats have an inhibiting effect

on digestive secretion and lessen the amount and activity of pepsin and hydrochloric acid necessary for the digestion of protein.

4. Use fats sparingly, as they inhibit the secretion of gastric juices, except avocado fats which delay the passage of the starch from the stomach into the intestine. However, when fats such as avocado or nuts are eaten with raw, green vegetables, their inhibiting effects on gastric secretion is counteracted and digestion proceeds normally.

5. Do not eat acid foods with proteins such as citrus fruits. Pineapples, tomatoes, strawberries and other acid foods, should not be eaten with nuts, cheese, eggs or meat.

6. Do not combine sweet foods with protein, starch or acid foods. The sugars in sweet foods should be free to leave the stomach within 20 minutes and are apt to ferment if digestion is delayed by mixing with other foods. Sugar and starch combinations cause additional problems because, when sugar is taken, the mouth quickly fills with saliva, but there are no enzymes, such as ptyalin, present.

7. Eat only one concentrated starch per meal. This rule is more important as a means of avoiding over-eating starches than avoiding a bad combination. Slightly starchy vegetables may be combined with more starchy vegetables, such as carrots and potatoes, but not with combination foods such as grains and legumes.

8. Acid fruit may be used with sub-acid fruits. This works best when combined with less sweet sub-acid fruit. Tomato should not be combined with sub-acid fruit, nor with any other kind of fruit.

9. Sub-acid fruit may be used with sweet fruit. It is best to use the sweeter varieties of sub-acid fruits when making this combination. For people with poor digestion, bananas are best eaten alone. Always remember that there are two jealous fruits: melon and banana. Never eat these with other fruits.

10. Combine fruit only with lettuce and celery, and never combine fruits and vegetables in one meal. Remember that these should be eaten at separate times.

One final piece of practical advice is to drink plenty of fluid, such as still-water, fruit and vegetable juices, and be careful with the use of spices and condiments.

It is impossible to overstress that never is diet more important than during pregnancy. There is a wise Chinese saying: 'Disease enters through the mouth'. The mother's responsibility for a healthy diet does not stop at the time of the baby's birth. The following article on baby foods was written by Jill Parking in the *Daily Express*, 17 April 1991:

Baby Food is a Bad Recipe
The news that many manufactured baby foods fail to give babies the nutrition they need has thrown parents into an agony of worry and guilt. A new report by the Food Commission came out with the startling result that to take in enough calories, a baby between eight and ten months old would need to eat seven or eight jars of baby food a day.

'Nutrition', the report from the independent food safety watchdog, may well force many parents into a rethink on how they feed their babies. Baby food manufacturers have attacked the report which found that 68 of the 172 branded foods tested failed to reach the minimum calorific value laid down by experts in infant nutrition. Another 38 out of 97 savoury meals tested were below standard protein levels. Artificial flavourings are used and meals are bulked out with water and thickeners. The report claims home-made baby food is cheaper, more convenient and far superior in terms of infant nutrition. But tinned and bottled foods have long been considered a godsend by mothers who are too busy to cook baby portions, or who fear getting it wrong. There's an assumption that the manufacturers are the experts and they must be right.

A recent newspaper article, written by Natalie Angier, on research into the remarkable powers of breast-milk and how it shapes our lives, reads as follows:

As scientists lately have struggled to learn exactly what human milk is made of, the list of ingredients has become so long that breast-feeding infants should be grateful their packages come without a food label. Beyond the proteins, minerals, vitamins, fats, and sugars needed for nourishment, there are antibodies in milk to help fend off infection during the early months, when the baby's own immune system is still too weak to work; growth factors thought to help in tissue development and maturation; and an abundance of hormones, neuropeptides, and natural opioids that may subtly shape the newborn's brain and behaviour. Now, researchers have found proof for what they have long suspected: not only does the breast extract potent hormones from the mother's blood and concentrate them in the milk (as research has shown often happens); it also generates some of these hormones itself, to ensure that a rich, yet precisely calibrated, supply of the compounds will end up in the infant's food. Scientists already knew that the important brain hormone gonadotropin, abbreviated GnRH, which has a stimulating influence, exists in human milk in concentrations far exceeding the levels seen in the mother's blood, a discrepancy suggesting that a nursing woman's breast-tissue generates the hormone on its own.

What exactly the hormone does for a suckling infant remains unclear, but researchers propose that it influences the development of the newborn's sex organs, forestalling their maturation until the offspring is ready for reproduction. It could also assist in the wiring of the brain regions in command of sexual behaviour. The new discovery highlights scientists' growing appreciation that the breast is not a passive udder designed simply to dispense calories to a baby, but an active gland which directs the course of the newborn's great unfolding.

It is suggested that the breast be thought of as the external counterpart of the placenta, picking up where the large, liver-like structure left off the task of ushering the infant towards physical and neurological completion. The placenta is already known to synthesise GnRH and deliver it to the foetus, just as the breast has now been shown to do. The placenta is responsible for regulating the growth and differentiation of an embryo. But, after birth, not all the organs of the infant are fully developed. As the brain is still growing, the breast could be doing a similar job to that of the placenta.

Analysing breast-milk, researchers have found the hormone melatonin, which is thought to help the body keep time and may enable the infant to know when it should eat. They have found oxytocin, a hormone associated with affiliative impulses, which may help initiate the onset of a loving bond between mother and infant. Various thyroid hormones have been found and it has been argued whether breast-feeding can alleviate and even prevent the symptoms of congenital hypothyroidism, a condition that can result in severe mental retardation. Bradykinin, a small hormone involved in the sensation of pain, has been seen and also endorphins, the body's natural painkillers. One researcher summed up human milk as 'an incredibly complicated substance'.

cow's milk or soya milk. In most cases a mother's milk is rarely disagreeable to her baby, but this is not always so with man-made infant formulas. An allergic reaction to milk is a fairly frequent occurrence nowadays, and can cause a lot of grief to both mother and baby unless it is recognised in good time. In such instances quite a number of my patients have been very satisfied with a substitute product called Nanny; a goat's milk infant food. This product is a nutritionally suitable alternative for use in the diet of those infants and children who experience difficulties in tolerating cow's milk proteins.

Ordinary unmodified goat's milk is unsuitable for infant feeding and is not recommended for infants under the age of six months. It is too concentrated in its protein and mineral content which imposes undue burdens on the infant kidneys. The nutrition formula Nanny is a goat's milk formula where these problems have been corrected, and which supplies all the vitamins and minerals in the recommended amounts for infant health and growth. It is sucrose-free, no glucose syrups have been added and its unique fat blend with increased levels of unsaturated fats is helpful to the baby's fat absorption, and consequently to its digestion. Because this formula lacks the homologue of heat stable allergen in cow's milk, it can be used successfully in place of the widely used cow's milk-based infant formulas for those infants and children with a sensitivity to cow's milk protein. Goat's milk casein has half the curd of cow's milk and is therefore easier to digest, making it a successful substitute for babies with minor digestive problems.

It is evident that, although human-milk formula is perfect, the protein in goat's milk compares well with that of human milk, particularly in respect of the amino acid composition. The few instances where human milk has a slightly higher level of amino acids are compensated for in the moderately higher total protein content of goat's milk formula. The excess of other amino acids can easily be converted into energy.

Another important factor is tyrosine, a sulpha amino acid not essential in adults, but now considered by some scientists to be essential for normal retinal formation and in platelet functions in infants. Since neither cow's nor goat's milk contains taurine, it has been added to this formula to mimic the level in human milk.

Returning to the subject of breast-feeding, I would like to quote some results obtained during a national survey:

In 1985, 64 per cent of mothers in Britain breast-fed their babies at birth. The highest rate, 74 per cent, was in London and the South East. The rate fell progressively when moving north, and the lowest rate of 48 per cent was in Scotland. Young mothers, and mothers in social classes IV and V, were the groups with the lowest rates of breast-feeding. By the sixth week, only 39 per cent of mothers were breast-feeding their babies. The most common reasons for giving up were said to be insufficient milk and sore nipples. Of the bottle-fed newborn babies, about 80 per cent were started on whey-dominant infant formulas. Use of casein-dominant formulas increased with age, so that, at four to five months, more than half the bottle-fed babies were given this type of formula.

The results of the 1985 survey show a slight trend towards a decline in breast-feeding when compared with a similar survey carried out in 1980:

In 1980, 30 per cent of first-time mothers said that they had decided how to feed their babies before they became pregnant. In subsequent pregnancies, even more mothers had decided how to feed their baby before becoming pregnant. In the same year, 10 per cent of first-time mothers had no ante-natal discussion about infant feeding.

Although the goat's milk is good, any animal milk loses the enzymes for digestion in processing. Therefore, all it succeeds in doing is taxing the body's energy, which can result in colds (as milk is highly mucus forming), wind, constipation, diarrhoea, stomach aches and colic. In some scientific tests it has been noted that when animal-milk protein is found in human milk, this can manifest itself in other conditions, resulting in an overweight baby or increasing the possibility of diseases.

At about the fourth month, the baby's digestive system is sufficiently developed to start on the gradual change to solids. The following schedule will give the mother of a young baby some idea of what solid foods can be gradually introduced, and when.

Baby's introduction to solid foods – this should begin at 3½–4 months

Time of Feed	Week 1	Week 2	Week 3	Week 4	Week 5	Week 6	Week 7	Week 8
Every four hrs. e.g. 6.00 a.m.	Milk (breast or dried fortified milk)	Milk	Milk	Milk	Milk	Milk	Milk	Milk
10.00 a.m.	Cereal 1 teasp. fortified cereal 1–2 tbsp. milk from feed	Cereal	Cereal	Cereal	Cereal	9.30 a.m. Cereal	9.00 a.m. Cereal Diluted fruit juice	8.30 a.m. Cereal Diluted fruit juice
	Milk	Milk	Milk	Milk	Milk	Milk	Milk	Milk
2.00 p.m.		Home-made soup purée (1 tbsp.)	Fruit purée (1 tbsp.)	Purée vegetables (1 tbsp.)	1.30 p.m. Mashed potato and gravy (1 tbsp.)	1.00 p.m. Milk pudding (1 tbsp.) Fruit purée	12.30 p.m. White fish in milk (1 tbsp.) Vegetable purée	12.00 p.m. Mashed potato Finely minced meat and gravy Vegetable purée
	Milk	Milk	Milk	Milk	Milk	Milk	Milk	Milk
6.00 p.m.			Home-made soup purée	Home-made soup purée	Home-made soup Fruit purée	5.30 p.m. Mashed potato and gravy Vegetable purée Milk vitamins	5.00 p.m. Mashed potato and little grated cheese Milk vitamins	4.30 p.m. Home-made soup Fruit purée Milk vitamins
	Milk vitamins	Milk vitamins	Milk vitamins	Milk vitamins	Milk vitamins	Milk	Milk	Milk
10.00 p.m.	Milk	Milk	Milk	Milk	Milk	Milk	Milk	Milk

Kitchen equipment – Sieve, wooden spoon, liquidiser, juice extractor, squeezer, fork, clean bowl, mincer, grater – will make your own foods into correct consistency for the baby.

Tinned, packet and jars of food are useful only if you have nothing suitable in the home. Try new foods at 10.00 a.m. or 2.00 p.m.

Prevent excessive weight gain – avoid chocolate, sweets, biscuits, rusks, honey, jam and squashes.

Vitamin supplements (added from four weeks) should be continued until two years old.

Never less than 20 oz. (1 pint) of milk should be given daily – dried fortified milk should be continued until one year old.

3

Vitamins, Minerals and Trace Elements

A while ago, Lord Walton, in a public statement, referred to the need for research into babies with a low birth-weight. The background to this statement was explained in an article in *Health Magazine*, 22 August 1993, stating that in the last 12 years more newborn babies had been lighter than normal, causing great concern, particularly with respect to the influence of alcohol or nicotine. Checks into those small babies confirmed the likely causes to be poor nutrition, influence of drugs, or a deficiency of B vitamins and/or folic acid. In a number of these cases problems of spina bifida or other neuro defects were diagnosed. Improper nutrition is not always recognised, but what came to light was that 47,000 babies born in England and Wales were below the normal birth-weight of approximately 7.5 lbs.

Unfortunately, not all babies are born perfect. Approximately one in every 100 babies born has a congenital disease, such as spina bifida, a cleft palate, or a harelip, and, of course, there must be a reason for this. It is thought that such conditions may result from one's pre-natal environment, or perhaps the cause is little more than a single cell slightly out of alignment at the moment of conception. The characteristics inherited by the baby from the parents can be detected in the structure of the cell. They are carried by the chromosomes, which are small bodies in the kernel of the cell, and determine the growth of the individual. Half the chromosomes are supplied by the sperm cell and half by the egg cell of the mother. These chromosomes group together and influence the development of the foetus. Some of these inherited characteristics will dominate others. They intrinsically affect the condition of the child and illnesses can be inherited in this way. However, not all illness or disease in a child is inherited. Sometimes a cell mutation can cause a spontaneous change. A cell mutation can affect the development process, damaging the foetus whilst it is still in the womb. In the first few months of the development of the foetus, while the organs are being formed, the foetus is still at risk. Drugs, irresponsible medication, or the mother coming into contact with a contagious disease, such as German measles, or a virus during the early stages of her pregnancy, are likely to affect the health of her unborn baby. The immunity of the mother plays a major role here, although it is not known to what extent. Earlier this century, before the discovery of antibiotics, syphilis had an enormous influence, and this often severely affected the health of the unborn child.

Any medication used during pregnancy should only be taken with the knowledge and approval of your doctor or practitioner. Failed, self-induced abortions often result in the birth of a malformed baby; a baby with vertebral, brain or heart problems. Spina bifida, one of the most frequently occurring of the congenital spinal diseases, can occur once or twice in every thousand babies. Not only is the alignment of the vertebrae defective, but the nerve cells in the core of the vertebrae remain under-developed and often become infected which can cause serious problems. Sometimes a symptom of spina bifida is hydrocephalus, which is an enlargement of the skull caused by fluid around the brain. Fortunately, this is less common nowadays. The cerebro-spinal fluid is of great importance to the brain and if this is impaired, severe physical handicap may result.

Another possible defective condition is a hole in the heart, and this is mostly dictated by conditions during the first ten weeks of the pregnancy. A baby suffering from cyanosis, a condition that is responsible for an oxygen deficiency in the blood, will appear slightly blue. The heart does not fully function and the blood flow to the lungs is interrupted. A hole in the dividing wall of the heart causes a narrowing of the blood vessels to the lungs and an oxygen blockage. This can, in later life, lead to a heart condition.

When either the father or mother have a deviation in their chromosomes, Down's syndrome can occur. In the case of a Down's syndrome baby there is an extra chromosome in the twenty-first pair of chromosomes so that the total number of chromosomes is 47 instead of 46. Elderly women present a higher risk of giving birth to a mongoloid baby than younger mothers, and such a condition is immediately apparent at birth. Extra chromosomes can cause different abnormalities, such as the Syndrome of Klinefelter, which can result in a number of genetic deviations, such as sterility.

Chromosomal inconsistencies can cause hermaphrodites, or typically, phenylketonuria, which can be treated by a low-protein diet. Such a child has a shortage of an enzyme that is important for protein assimilation. In such cases diet is vital in order for the child to grow normally, and nowadays conditions such as a harelip or a cleft palate can usually be successfully rectified by surgery. Hormone deficiencies can also be the cause of genetic deviations, but, luckily, in our day and age these can usually be solved if discovered at an early stage.

Prevention, however, is better than cure, and therefore it is helpful if we look carefully at what can be safely taken to help certain conditions. Is there, for instance, proof that the use of extra vitamin C can help to avoid cot deaths? Many pregnant women or women who want to become pregnant have asked my advice on this. If they had had a miscarriage before they would be willing to do anything at all to become pregnant, and carry the baby full-term. In many cases all that was necessary was a dietary change and some supplementary vitamins, minerals and trace elements. If I thought it might be helpful, I might also prescribe a safe homoeopathic or herbal remedy, and very often these patients had no problems during the subsequent pregnancy. Women who had experienced complications such as rejection of the foetus, have also benefited from similar remedies. Never is it more important than during pregnancy to eat a wholesome diet with plenty of fresh fruits, vegetables, nuts, rice, and so on. This will help the pregnant mother not only to carry her baby full term but also to give birth to a healthy child.

Immunity or resistance to disease is of great importance and dependent on the three sources of energy: food, water and air. Sadly, these energy sources are not what they used to be and some extra help is necessary. I have already briefly referred to deficiencies of the B vitamins and folic acid, and recent reports have also mentioned pantothenic acid, and how important it is to ensure that the body receives these substances. Yet another study group proposes that even a small supplement of the vitamin may be enough to give that little extra boost. Scientists continue to investigate the secrets of vitamins and an article in the *Daily Telegraph* on Wednesday, 10 April 1991, written by the science editor, discusses the complexity of vitamins and, in particular, the B12 vitamin:

Scientists are close to uncovering how nature manages to make the most complex vitamins after a discovery by an Anglo-French team. It is a breakthrough that has led to a change in direction of an intensive research effort that has already taken 10 years, the 150th Annual Chemical Congress in London was told yesterday. Vitamin B12 is a large, complicated molecule that assists essential biochemical processes, but cannot be made in the body so it must be taken up from food. A person who is unable to absorb the vitamin suffers pernicious anaemia, which slows the rate at which healthy red blood cells form, preventing oxygen from being transported efficiently around the body. But the vitamin is made by some micro-organisms in a highly efficient way. 'The challenge is to find out how these bugs make this fantastic molecule. And they do it, of course, by superb chemistry,' said Prof. Alan Battersby, of Cambridge University. 'Once you know how it is done, you can engineer the organism to do a better job.'

Prof. Battersby reported how he, working with the Centre de Recherche de Vitry, Rhone-Poulenc Sante, France, had discovered a key intermediate in the manufacture of the vitamin in the micro-organism, a process that takes tens of steps. 'You start with A and are going to B and do not know which way to go. It is like finding a signpost halfway between them,' he said. They did it by understanding the genetics and tracing the fate of carbon atoms by using carbon isotopes. 'The result has changed the direction of the research,' he said. Called precorrin-6, the intermediate is a large molecule consisting of 52 carbon atoms, 70 hydrogen atoms, four nitrogens and 16 oxygens, though it is not as large as the vitamin B12.

I can understand the confusion on the subject of vitamins. Many people think that if they eat enough fruit fresh and vegetables and sufficient wholesome food, then additional vitamins should not be necessary. It should be understood that the human body consists of millions of cells and in each cell multiple biochemical reactions occur every second. Vitamins participate in these reactions and must be present in proper proportions in order for the body to function correctly. Unfortunately, nowadays people often do not get the right quantities of these vitamins through their food. Things were different when people used to eat more roughage and a more natural diet which contained the vitamins they needed. The science of nutrition has evolved quite rapidly and has discovered the value of vitamins and other dietary substances.

We have known for centuries that a vitamin C deficiency is likely to result in scurvy, but this vitamin also plays a very important role in the effectiveness of the immune system. Unfortunately, one of the side-effects of an allergy is that it can easily cause a deficiency. I was astounded by the mother who brought her twelve-year-old to see me, having visited all kinds of allergy clinics and, following their advice, cut out all the apparently offending foodstuffs. Imagine my amazement when, in 1992, I was presented with a child suffering from scurvy as a result of a vitamin deficiency. It just shows how careful we must be. The recommendation levels on vitamin bottles are a guideline only, and I would advise that, especially during pregnancy, a woman discusses the requirement of vitamin supplements with her doctor, practitioner or midwife.

It is surprising how often deficiencies are still discovered in our affluent society. I have come across deficiencies of the vitamins A, C, B1, B2, B6 and B12, magnesium, iron, calcium and selenium, as well as other minerals and trace elements, and I can assure you that such defiencies do not happen overnight. This is a gradual process and one should be aware of the symptoms in order to recognise a deficiency. An understanding of vitamin, mineral and trace elements deficiencies can be achieved by reading up on the subject. A deficiency can usually be corrected by a change in diet.

There are additional risk factors when women are pregnant or lactating because of extra demands on the body by the foetus or the baby. Pregnant and nursing mothers have an increased need for all vitamins, especially A, C, B6 and B12, pantothenic acid, folic acid and the minerals iron and calcium. Dietary management then is even more important and the concept should be considered in its entirety. If a pregnant woman has been dieting and her food intake has been reduced, it is important that she take extra vitamins. The same advice goes for drug-taking, drinking or smoking mothers. In this respect I must also mention the use of 'the pill'. The oral contraceptive pill lowers the absorption of vitamins, and increases the need for B6 and folic acid.

Moderate smoking reduces the blood vitamin C levels by 20 per cent and heavy smoking by 40 per cent. This may result in a more rapid vitamin turnover than in non-smokers, and so may impair the immune defence system. A research group has carefully investigated this and the results were published in a booklet distributed by the pharmaceutical company, Roche:

Potential risk factors were listed as follows:
• Dieting: adolescents and adult women
• Decreased caloric needs: the elderly
• Meal skipping: adolescents, adult women, adult men and the elderly

- Unbalanced diet: adolescents, adult women, adult men and the elderly
- Heavy drinking: adult women, adult men and the elderly
- Nutrient losses in food preparation: children, adolescents, pregnant and nursing women, adult women, adult men and the elderly
- Chronic medication: adult women, adult men and the elderly
- Heavy smoking: adolescents, adult women, adult men and the elderly
- Periods of increased needs: children, adolescents, pregnant and nursing women

Although the daily food intake should provide adequate vitamins and minerals, we know that today's eating habits make it less likely that these needs are being met. The enrichment of staple and convenience foods in recent years removed many of the vitamin requirements. Moreover, supplements offer additional benefits by preventing the development of other problems.

Most vitamin manufacturers state on the labels of their packaging if they are suitable during pregnancy. Generally speaking, vitamins are safe even if taken in doses above the recommended daily dietary levels, but there are exceptions, and it is definitely not a case of the more the better. It should be emphasised that with excessive intake of vitamins A and D adverse effects are possible. The following table provides the reader with a basic knowledge of vitamin requirements (see pages 44 and 45).

Vitamins

Vitamins are essential to health, but a little basic knowledge will help you to understand their role. Vitamins function closely with enzymes and together they control biochemical reactions within the cells and tissues of the body. With the exception of vitamin D, our requirement for most of the other vitamins relies on us extracting these vital nutrients from our diet. A well-balanced diet, with plenty of fresh fruit and uncooked vegetables, carefully prepared, can provide all we need, but up to 90 per cent of available vitamins can be lost for food by either peeling, freezing or cooking.

There are two main groups of vitamins: water soluble ones, such as the B vitamins and vitamin C, which are not stored in the body and must be regularly replaced; and fat soluble ones, such as vitamins A, D and E, which are stored in the body.

Vitamin A occurs naturally in two forms; as retinol and as carotene. Retinol is preformed vitamin A and is only found in foods of animal origin, such as liver and fish oil, and is produced by these animals from carotene. Carotene is found in green vegetables and carrots and our bodies are able to convert it into vitamin A. Over 90 per cent of the body's vitamin A is stored in the liver. Vitamin A is needed for:

- healthy skin and tissues
- the mucous membranes of the lungs, throat, nose and mouth
- a healthy immune system
- healthy, moist eyes and vision
- the formation of blood, bones and teeth

The B vitamins are known as a 'complex'. They occur together in natural sources and their uses in the body dovetail. Most people prefer to take a B-complex which supplies all the B vitamins together, but if you decide to take any of the single Bs on their own, remember that, in the long term, you should take a B-complex as well. The best sources of B vitamins are foods which today seem less popular than they were, such as brewer's yeast, liver and wholegrains. Since B vitamins are water soluble, they are not stored in the body and must be regularly replaced. B vitamins are needed for:

- their role in releasing energy from food
- maintaining a healthy digestive system
- the normal functioning of the nerves and brain
- the metabolism of fats and proteins
- maintaining healthy skin, hair, eyes, mouth and mucous membranes
- repair and regeneration of the liver
- the production of red blood cells and haemoglobin

Vitamin B6 is needed for:

- the metabolism of essential fatty acids and amino acids
- the health of the nervous system
- the immune system
- the skin
- the production of vital chemicals such as the brain and mood hormone, Serotonin
- the maintenance of the body's water balance

Unused B6 leaves the body in the urine within eight hours so regular replenishment is important.

Vitamin	Functions	Food sources high in vitamins	Factors influencing stability	Range of Recommended Dietary Allowances*	Classical deficiency symptoms
A (Retinol)	Essential for normal growth, healthy skin, eyes, teeth, gums and hair.	Yellow vegetables, liver, eggs, milk, butter, margarine.	Light, heat, oxidising agents.	4000-5000 IU (International Units)	Night-blindness, lowered resistance to infections, blindness (xerophthalmia).
D	For strong teeth and bones. Helps the body utilise calcium and phosphorus.	Fortified milk, margarine, egg yolk, tuna, salmon.	Light, heat, oxidising agents.	200-400 IU	Bone deformities (rickets and osteomalacia).
E (Tocopherol)	Helps the formation and functioning of red blood cells, muscle and other tissues. Protects essential fatty acids.	Vegetable oils, whole grain cereals, vegetables, nuts.	Light, heat, oxidising agents.	12-15 IU	Wasting of the muscles (dystrophy), neurological disorders (neuropathy).
K	Necessary for normal blood clotting.	Leafy green vegetables.	Light.	50-140 mcg** (micrograms)	Haemorrhages, mainly in newborn infants.
B₁ (Thiamin)	Helps to get energy from food by promoting proper metabolism of sugars and fatty acids. For correct functioning of heart and nervous system.	Pork, whole grains, lamb, beef, poultry.	Light, heat, humidity.	1.0-1.5 mg (milligrams)	Nervous disorder, beriberi.
B₂ (Riboflavin)	Necessary for healthy skin. Functions in the body's use of carbohydrates, proteins and fats. Helps release energy to cells.	Milk, cheese, meat, eggs, whole grains, leafy green vegetables.	Light.	1.2-1.7 mg	Changes in skin and mucous membranes.
Niacin PP	Involved in energy-producing reactions in cells. Aids the nervous system.	Meat, fish, wheat, whole grains.	None.	13-19 mg	Nervous disorders, diarrhoea, skin changes (dermatitis) pellagra.
Pantothenic acid	Required for the metabolism of proteins, fats and carbohydrates, and for the formation of certain hormones. Functions in the regeneration of tissues.	Found in nearly all foods.	Heat, humidity.	4-7 mg**	Nervous and intestinal disorders.

Vitamin	Functions	Food sources high in vitamins	Factors influencing stability	Range of Recommended Dietary Allowances*	Classical deficiency symptoms
B6 (Pyridoxine)	Essential for proper utilisation of proteins. Aids in the formation of red blood cells and correct functioning of the nervous system.	Lean meat, leafy green vegetables, whole grain cereals, bananas.	Light.	1.8-2.2 mg	Nervous disorders, convulsions, anaemia.
B12 (Cyano-cobalamin)	Helps prevent certain forms of anaemia. Assists in the formation of red blood cells.	Meat, fish, eggs, milk.	Light, humidity.	3 mcg	Nervous disorders, pernicious anaemia.
Folic acid (BC)	Aids in the formation of cells, especially red blood cells. Helps maintain functions of the intestinal tract and prevent certain forms of anaemia.	Leafy green vegetables, yellow fruits and vegetables.	Light, oxidising agents.	400 mcg	Intestinal disorders, anaemia.
Biotin (H)	Involved in the formation of fatty acids and production of energy. Essential to many chemical systems in the body.	Egg yolk, green vegetables, milk.	None.	100-200 mcg**	Skin changes (dermatitis), loss of hair.
C (Ascorbic acid)	Helps keep bone, teeth and blood vessels healthy. Important in the formation of collagen, a protein that helps support body structures. Aids in the absorption of iron. Plays a role in the body's self-defence mechanism.	Citrus fruits, potatoes, broccoli, cabbage, tomatoes.	Heat, humidity, oxidising agents.	50-60 mcg	Lowered resistance to infection, sore gums, haemorrhages, scurvy.

* According to the Food and Nutrition Board of the National Academy of Sciences National Research Council (1980), designed 'for the maintenance of good nutrition for practically all healthy people in the USA'. The ranges apply to persons over 10 years of age. Recommended Daily Dietary Allowances for expectant or nursing mothers may exceed the indicated maxima.

** Estimated Safe and Adequate Daily Intake (National Academy of Sciences, USA, 1980).

Folic acid appears in many forms in the diet although not all of them can be fully utilised by the human body, and in recent surveys, folic acid was shown to be one of the nutrients most often missing from our diets. The best sources of folic acid are green, leafy vegetables, liver and brewer's yeast, although 65 per cent of the folic acid in these foods can be lost during refining and processing. Folic acid is needed for:

- the formation of iron for carrying haemoglobin which is required by red blood cells and for the metabolism of RNA and DNA (the nucleic acids at the source of cell life)
- its role in the performance of the liver in the production of digestive acid
- a healthy appetite
- periods of unusual bio-activity such as pregnancy and growth

Vitamin B12 is found mainly in animal-based foods such as meat, but some experts are not convinced that it is in forms which the human body can absorb. B12 is often chosen as a regular supplement by vegetarians and vegans. It is essential for the normal metabolism of nerve tissue and for a healthy myelin sheath, the insulation of our nerves.

Vitamin C is a unique nutrient, known to be involved either directly or indirectly in at least 300 biochemical pathways in the body. Unlike most animals, we can no longer synthesise it and so we rely instead on a constant supply every day from our food. Our daily requirement of Vitamin C is higher than for any other water-soluble vitamin. It is highly unstable and easily destroyed by the process of storing, peeling, freezing and cooking and so it is not always possible to be sure how much is taken in the diet. Vitamin C is needed for:

- the production of collagen, a tough fibrous protein which is an integral part of skin, tendons, bones, gums, teeth and blood vessels
- its protective role as a free radical scavenger with anti-oxidant properties
- a healthy immune system
- the maintenance of healthy bones, teeth and gums
- helping to maintain normal blood fat and cholesterol levels
- the growth and repair of tissue
- fat metabolism

Vitamin D can either be ingested in food or manufactured by the body from sunlight on the skin. Vitamin D is needed for the proper absorption of calcium, and phosphorus to form healthy bones and teeth. It is a popular choice for those who are housebound.

Vitamin E is fat soluble and is both stored and transported around the body dissolved in fats, whereas the other important anti-oxidant nutrient, vitamin C, is restricted to the water-based parts of our tissues. Vitamin E protects polyunsaturated fats from being oxidised into saturated fat, and so protects all membranes including those in blood-vessel walls. The protective role of vitamin E has placed it at the centre of worldwide research (along with vitamin C and beta carotene), into the relationship between the intake of nutrients and our long-term health. Vitamin E also plays a role in the health of capillary walls and the strength of blood vessels, the health of the reproductive system and the maintenance of healthy skin.

Minerals

Every mineral in our body has come from the food that we have eaten. Minerals originate from the soil and are taken up by plants which are then eaten by us. Vitamins, on the other hand, do not come from the soil but are instead synthesised by plants. Minerals are often metals such as iron and zinc and, although they cannot usually be destroyed by cooking, they can easily be lost from our food by peeling, by boiling and, in the case of rice and cereals, by polishing. Also, modern-day diets of high energy, fatty foods are known to be low in minerals.

Minerals are split into two main groups; macrominerals and trace elements, the only difference being the amount required by our bodies. For example, a 70 kg man has 1.7 kilos of calcium (a macromineral) in his body but only 50 mg of the trace element iodine. Both are essential but one is present at levels 34,000 times the level of the other. The most common minerals are:

Macrominerals	Trace Elements
Calcium	Zinc
Magnesium	Selenium
Sodium	Iodine
Chlorine	Iron
Phosphorus	Manganese
Potassium	Chromium

Iron is one of the most common nutrients to be deficient among women, as the iron contained in red blood cells is lost during menstruation. Iron plays a vitally important role, since it is involved

47

in the transport of oxygen around our bodies. Iron is a component of some proteins both in the blood and in the muscles. It is most readily obtained from meat, particularly liver, so vegetarians and anyone who eats little red meat should be careful with their iron intake, and ought to consider a supplement.

Zinc is a trace element involved in hundreds of metabolic reactions and is also a co-factor of more than 80 enzymes in the body. Up to 20 per cent of the zinc in our bodies is present in the skin where it plays a role in maintaining the complexion. Zinc is required for:

- healthy growth through its role in the synthesis of DNA and protein
- maintaining the immune system
- the balance of blood sugar through insulin
- maintaining a healthy liver
- maintaining our sense of smell, taste and vision
- the healthy functioning of the reproductive organs particularly in men, since it is a component of semen

Many nutritionists believe that more people find it difficult to obtain enough zinc in their diet than any other mineral because of modern agriculture and food processing methods. Foods rich in zinc include red meat, eggs and fish. Vegetables contain lower amounts of zinc and sometimes this is bound up in indigestible fibre, effectively reducing the usefulness of vegetables as a source of zinc. This is why vegetarians and vegans often choose to take a zinc supplement as should smokers, the elderly and athletes; the latter because zinc is lost in sweat.

Calcium and magnesium are needed for both formation and health because the calcium is used structurally, whilst the magnesium helps to guide the calcium into the bones and away from the soft tissues of the body. It is this relationship between the two minerals that has led many nutritionists to recommend that food supplements should contain a 2:1 ratio of calcium to magnesium. A sensible amount to supplement the diet with would be 500 mg of calcium and 250 mg of magnesium, although menopausal women may choose to double this.

Trace Mineral Complex is a formula that contains all the most important minerals, including small amounts of calcium and magnesium for their possible role in helping with the absorption of the other minerals. A high-potency combination of this formula is called Mega Mineral Complex. Both products are available from Nature's Best who have a very extensive line of vitamin and mineral supplements which I have worked with for many years. I know their products and recommendations to be safe, but I must, however, emphasise that pregnant women should not take any amino acids.

The most common conditions during pregnancy are constipation, indigestion, heartburn, toxaemia, urinary infections, and blood circulatory problems, such as cramp, varicose veins, haemorrhoids. In some of these instances additional vitamins, minerals and trace elements can be very helpful. Varicose veins, partly because of their external appearance, can cause women great distress. These are often caused by a hindrance to the transport of blood through the veins because of ineffective valves, which regulate the reverse flow of the blood, or because of degeneration of the veins. Varicose veins generally occur in the lower legs, although they can also appear in other parts of the body. The symptoms are swollen blue veins, heaviness, tiredness, and a painful sensation in the legs, especially towards the end of the day. Swollen ankles and feet, and sensitivity in the veins can occur during menstruation. In later life, it may be symptomised by eczema, a brown discoloration of the skin, and even sores.

Varicose veins often appear during or after pregnancy, in cases of obesity, or in those people – men and women alike – whose job requires them to be on their feet for long periods of time. If the cause is obesity, the obvious answer is that the person concerned should lose weight. In order to prevent varicose veins occurring: take sufficient physical exercise, and avoid sitting or standing for long spells. Never sit with the legs crossed, avoid high blood pressure and, when sleeping or taking a rest, raise the legs. Any treatment for varicose veins should be directed towards the improvement of the circulation and the strengthening of the vascular system. You should avoid salt, products containing white flour, and any fattening foods. Try to eat more wholemeal products, pineapple juice, grapefruit juice, currants, raisins and grapes. Twice a day take ten drops of Hyperisan before meals and also twice a day, three tablets of Urticalcin after meals.

Constipation, the slow elimination of waste from the bowels causing the stools to be hard, is not uncommon in pregnancy. However, if you are not pregnant, the cause could be a bowel obstruction or infection, diverticulitis (inflammation, commonly in the colon), irregular bowel movements, changes in diet or environment, dehydration causing thickness in faeces, lack of physical exercise or nervous tension. The treatment for constipation should consist of a change in dietary habits, thus stimulating waste elimination and avoiding dehydration. Chewing half a teaspoon of Linoforce twice a day will usually help to regulate the bowel movements.

The painful condition of haemorrhoids is caused by a swelling of the veins in the rectum and around the anus. Most likely causes are lack of physical exercise, chronic constipation, obesity, pregnancy, high blood pressure, vascular disease or weakness. Symptoms are swelling and heaviness around the anus, occasional slight bleeding in the stools, itchiness and burning sensation of the anal area. To treat this condition an improvement must be made in the circulatory system; dietary changes will avoid constipation and strengthen the vascular system. In the diet avoid salt, products containing white flour, hard-boiled eggs, excess meat, coffee, sugar and chocolate. The diet should contain bran, raw vegetables and fruit, raisins, grapes, and anything known to improve bowel movements. Increased fluid intake is also important. Useful remedies are Hyperisan (ten drops twice daily before meals) and Urticalcin (three tablets twice daily after meals).

High blood pressure can be caused by stress and nervous tension, smoking, too much salt in the food, kidney dysfunction, narrowing of the veins, oral contraceptives, obesity and lack of physical exercise. It should be remembered that high blood pressure may also be hereditary. The symptoms of high blood pressure are not easily noted and this condition is usually only diagnosed during a general check-up. Symptoms may express themselves as headaches, nervousness, sleeplessness, nose-bleeds, shortage of breath and oedema, or fluid retention.

High blood pressure can be treated by regulating the elimination of fluid from the body, strengthening the vascular system and reducing nervous tension. It is important to recognise that high blood pressure increases the risk of heart and vascular conditions, a brain haemorrhage or even kidney disease. Take more physical exercise and avoid stress. Make sure you are not overweight. Please remember that diuretics, which are often prescribed to help the elimination of fluid from the body, can also cause an excessive loss of potassium and magnesium, the two minerals that help keep the blood pressure down. The best dietary advice to maintain healthy blood pressure is to drastically reduce one's intake of salt, sugar, coffee, alcohol, meat and spices. Make sure to include potassium-rich foods, such as bananas, fruit juices, dried apricots, potatoes, raisins, figs, kiwi fruits, tomato juice and brown rice. Take three garlic capsules at night and fifteen drops of Arterioforce before meals.

Over the years, in the treatment of pregnant women and in my own family, I have become aware of many problems that can occur, but I have also seen the tremendous benefit of an improved diet, including a much easier pregnancy without sickness, an easier birth and faster recovery, a healthier baby at birth and, for both mother and baby, a better immune system. I have already mentioned the problems that can result from alcohol, smoking and drug abuse. Pay attention to the biblical advice in the book of Judges, given by a messenger of God, telling Samson's mother that she was about to conceive and would give birth to a son. The message includes the advice that she should not consume wine, or any other fermented drink. Very sound advice indeed. Alcohol has brought with it tremendous problems and fermented drinks are thought to be a primary reason for the increase in the occurrence of *Candida albicans*.

The World Health Organisation has done a great deal of research on this and cites a number of environmental hazards. No alcohol during pregnancy is the only safe limit. Smoking is another hazard, and the 43 per cent of children whose mothers are smokers in turn suffer from blood disorders, respiratory infections, bladder and kidney problems, and skin conditions is very sad. Both father and mother should consider this statement and stop smoking. I know that this is easier said than done, but there are many ways of getting help with this.

It is well known that any drug treatment, unless absolutely necessary, should be avoided during pregnancy.

Again, I would remind the reader that your sugar intake should be very low. Not only is sugar bad, but the moment it touches the tongue, it diminishes the effects of vitamins, minerals and trace elements. During pregnancy, when the risk of becoming diabetic or hypoglycaemic (having low blood sugar) is increased, an imbalance in the blood sugar-level makes it even more important to cut down the intake of sugar to no more than the essential requirement.

4

Homoeopathy

I work with and talk about homoeopathy daily and so I want to take this opportunity to summarise some of the theoretical and practical applications of homoeopathy. I believe that although the principle is generally accepted, homoeopathy may seem impractical when compared with conventional Western medicine. This does not negate the validity of a healing system which regards all symptoms as part of a larger holistic body. Homoeopathy works with us, not against us. It assists our innate intelligence and manifestation of good health and, as homoeopathy is based on the application of minute doses of specific substances, this form of medicine does not pose a problem during pregnancy.

Homoeopathy emerged as a highly systematic medical science through the efforts of a German physician and pharmacist, Samuel Hahnemann. In the nineteenth century, Dr Samuel Hahnemann, founder of homoeopathy, believed that remedies, which in large doses would create a particular set of symptoms, when taken in minute doses could actually relieve those symptoms. Strictly speaking, homoeopathy is a system of totally natural medicines, yet it can only temporarily improve symptoms which are caused and aggravated by continual exposure to personal, physical and emotional stress.

Hahnemann used the Latin phrase *similia similibus curentur* – like cures like. His methods are based on the principle that substances, when taken in a small dose, stimulate the organism to heal that which they cause in overdose. The medical system he devised was to be referred to as homoeopathy, derived from the Greek words *homoeo*, meaning similar, and *pathos*, for suffering or disease. This system of medical treatment is based on the theory that certain diseases can be cured with small doses of drugs which, in a healthy person and in large doses, would produce symptoms like those of the disease. This dispensable system is not all-inclusive but is applicable to many situations.

Hahnemann discovered that a substance which can mimic symptoms, can also help to cure a person. He came to a revolutionary understanding of symptoms instead of assuming that symptoms represent illogical, improper or unhealthy responses which should be treated with drugs or by surgery. Hahnemann learned that symptoms are positive, adaptive responses to the variety of stresses the body experiences and that symptoms represent the body's best efforts to heal itself. He believed that man has brought imbalance into a world which was once completely balanced, intelligent and supreme.

Dr Samuel Hahnemann began to experiment with the size of the doses to see how little medicine he could give to still cause a sustained healing response or healing crisis. After years of persistent and intensive study he found a method of diluting substances that kept the toxic properties at a minimum but magnified the potential for cure. He called this pharmaceutical process 'potentization' or 'succussion'. He did not want to follow the rest of the world's methods of treating symptoms. He wanted to treat the problem. When lecturing, I sometimes use the parable that if the church is on fire and the bells are ringing, it is possible to stop the ringing of the bells, but unless the water hose is activated, the fire will continue to rage. It is the same if one has a headache: this is an alarm bell indicating that somewhere in the body there is something wrong. It is possible to take a painkiller to stop the ringing of the bells, but the fire still goes on.

Symptoms accompany a disease or a condition, and symptoms are evidence of that disease, but treating symptoms is like killing the messenger bringing bad news. Because Hahnemann wanted to treat the body as a whole, a holistic system, his aim was to treat mind, body and spirit. The basic philosophy of holistic medicine is the belief that man has three bodies: a physical, a mental and an emotional body, and unless these are all considered in the treatment, there can be no proper cure. With this principle in mind it becomes clear that as the result of a deeper disturbance or an imbalance in a person, of which symptoms are simply the outward manifestation, their disease is a blockage in the flow of energy between these three bodies. This totality of symptoms can also be seen as an expression of the 'vital force', a dynamic energy of existence which animates everything that we call life. It is this vital force and its healing mechanism which are stimulated by homoeopathic remedies and this naturopathic therapy is used to release the blockage in the vital force. The four main principles Hahnemann adhered to were:

1. not to kill the good in the body when we try to kill the bad
2. that the healing crisis is most important in every illness and disease
3. to treat the harmony between mind, body and spirit – a life force so easily influenced, both positively and negatively
4. that the cause must be found

It could often be quite difficult to trace the underlying cause of an illness. Degenerative disease, for example, could easily be a late after-effect of some illness that had occurred during one's younger years which had not been correctly treated. A healing crisis is very important and my grandmother, who was a competent naturopath, always maintained that if a patient had a fever, the chances of treating that person successfully would be greatly increased. What she meant was that an increase in temperature enables the body to shed the malevolent influence, rather than allowing it to remain inside the body.

A miasma is a left-over from previous inflammations, viruses or infections, and homoeopathy is one of the most wonderful tools for clearing these miasmas once they have been identified, or for overcoming conditions in the body which have been inherited from previous generations. I have often suggested that women who want to become pregnant should have a blood test to see if there is any sign of a miasma. With the help of a homoeopathic remedy, such a condition could then be cured before they become pregnant. It is actually very important to have such miasmas cleared, as it is now suspected that multiple sclerosis, for example, may well be the result of a very severe condition of measles that was not correctly treated or brought to a crisis situation. For example, ME – Myalgic Encephalomyelitis – is suspected to be caused by the left-overs of glandular fever that was suppressed by antibiotics. It does no good to suppress illness or disease; it must be brought out of the body, and that is what homoeopathy is all about. The more natural the treatment of former illnesses, the better.

The vital force Hahnemann spoke about is the energy flow that can be affected by influences from the past. Yet, a minute dose of a homoeopathic remedy, as soon as it touches the tongue, may create a vibration in the body which can cause a radical change. Over the years I have seen some unusual cases where a minimal dose of a homoeopathic remedy caused the reaction or vibration in the body necessary to clear a specific condition.

I have no doubt whatsoever as to the effectiveness of homoeopathic treatment. Despite numerous attacks on the validity of the homoeopathic principle, I am convinced that it has managed to stand the test of time. It has been shown to meet the need for more economical and non-toxic therapy. It encompasses all areas of medical care: prevention, acute care and chronic diseases. Because they are safe, homoeopathic remedies are used throughout the world as they were in the past, moreover they can usually be combined with other forms of treatment. Sometimes homoeopathic remedies are alcohol-based, and if this is seen as a problem, the alcohol can be evaporated by leaving the remedy to stand for one minute in a glass of warm water. Another practical point to remember is not to use tap-water. It is better to use distilled or bottled water, as tap-water very often contains certain chemicals.

Modern homoeopathy owes a great deal to Samuel Hahnemann. In his early research he noted that a medicine called Cinchona, used at that time to treat malaria, provoked similar symptoms in otherwise healthy people. This discovery led to a great deal of detailed research. A very simple example is that when one peels an onion we get tears, a water discharge, or the symptoms of a cold. The same applies to the principle of homoeopathy. Changes in the body, such as pregnancy, when mind, body and soul are involved, can cause reactions; it can cause problems with digestion, heartburn or acidity.

There are safe homoeopathic medicines for indigestion, nausea and sickness, and one I have prescribed successfully for many years, even to pregnant women, is Nux vomica. The remedy helps to settle the digestive tracts, the veins and the arteries which are becoming too compressed by the expanding uterus.

Diabetes is not uncommon in pregnancy and, although it usually passes when the pregnancy is over, it requires careful monitoring as the risks during pregnancy and thereafter are much higher than usual. Diabetes Complex, as the name indicates, is a complex remedy; in other words, it is based on homoeopathic and herbal principles. Ten drops of this twice a day eases this condition. The dietary supplement Molkosan, which is derived from milk whey, is also effective. Or you can take on my grandmother's advice: shell one pound of walnuts and use the nuts in salads. Boil the shells in one pint of water for at least 20 minutes and dispose of the shells, retaining the fluid. Keep this in a cool place and drink a small glass of this extract every day. This is safe and very effective.

Breast discomfort during pregnancy is also a frequent complaint and if the breasts feel hard and tense Bryonia 6C can be used safely. If there is only mild discomfort, I would advise Conium 6C.

I remember the case of a young woman who confided in me that she was desperately trying to become pregnant and, during our conversation, I learned that as a child she had been very ill with German measles. Following my advice she took a nosode – Rubella 30C – which had a strong reaction, and I advised her to wait a while before trying to fall pregnant. I saw her at intervals during this time and gradually the miasmas from the German measles were cleared. After a trouble-free pregnancy she gave birth to a healthy baby.

Another common problem is a disturbed sleep pattern during pregnancy. The mother-to-be often complains that heartburn, the weight and awkwardness of a heavier body, and the need for more frequent visits to the bathroom cause her to wake more often during the night. Homoeopathic remedies such as Coffea 30C, Ignatia or Aconite are all completely safe to take and help to overcome these temporary troublesome side-effects.

Emotional disturbances are not unusual during pregnancy, and are often due to entering a previously unknown stage in life. There are a number of homoeopathic remedies that can be safely taken and some, which I have prescribed successfully over the years, are Aconite 30C, Ignatia 30C and Hamamilla 30C. You may rest assured that these remedies will not cause any harm to the baby. Sometimes I advise an emotionally tense mother-to-be, depending on her character, to take Pulsatilla 30C; this will also help to relieve any attacks of nausea she may experience. If the nausea is accompanied by sickness and dizziness, Nux vomica D4 is a very useful remedy. This can be used for dizziness, irritation and sensitivity to noise and light. Ipecacuanha D3 – ten drops three times a day – helps many patients who suffer from frequent sickness, especially if sputum is present. Tabacum D4 – ten drops three times a day before meals – is very helpful, and the benefits are greater still if the person takes plenty of fresh air.

Fortunately, severe toxaemia is rarely seen these days and regular antenatal care is certainly helping to keep it under control. This condition can occur during pregnancy, but often disappears after the birth of the baby. It can be detected very quickly in the early stages of pregnancy when it can be prevented from getting any worse. In a severe form the mother's blood can become poisoned and fits can occur. This is just one of the reasons for regular attendance at the antenatal clinic where blood pressure, urine, swelling ankles and body weight are regularly checked. Doctors and midwives are very alert to any signs of toxaemia and early recognition is the best way to avoid this rare condition.

Bearing in mind that protection is better than cure, a number of my patients have followed the advice in the Homoeopathic Pregnancy Programme, devised by a valued colleague, Dr Frank McConnachie from Belfast. This programme gives women the best protection possible before and during the birth:

The Homoeopathic Pregnancy Programme

Caulophyllum 30 (pills)
Take two doses, morning and evening, on alternate days, commencing *two months* prior to date of delivery.

Arnica 30 (tablets)
This remedy may be used at any time throughout pregnancy for the relief of soreness, tiredness and stretching of tissues, but should be taken daily for *two weeks* prior to date of delivery.

Bellis Perennis 12X (powders)
After the delivery take one powder daily for *four days* together with a daily dose of Arnica 30.

Calendula Mother Tincture
Twelve drops in one cup of warm, sterile water is useful for swabbing the perineal area after delivery.

Calendula Ointment
This will assist healing if spread lightly on any irritation.

Suck or chew pillules or tablets between meals – do not swallow with water. Tip the dose onto the lid of the bottle and transfer to the mouth. Similarly, the powders should be put directly onto the tongue and allowed to dissolve in the mouth – no water should be taken.

5

Herbal Medicine

Herbal medicine or, as it is called nowadays, phytotherapy, was always my favourite subject during my studies. I developed a great love for this subject and I have studied it a great deal. Hence, I know most plants, leaves and herbs by their common and Latin names, and, over the years, I have continued to study their scientific values and their medical and remedial properties. Even today whenever I get the opportunity to visit other parts of the world I add to this knowledge. When I was in the bush in Australia I realised how much there was I did not know. At the cost of billions of dollars we have sent men to the moon, but very little research has taken place into God's gift of nature. In a very busy career I have little time for hobbies, but I have always set aside time to study and further develop my interests in the characteristics and the properties of herbs and plants.

It is wonderful to recognise the design pattern in a herb and relate this to a possible medicinal remedy. Every time I learn about a new variety of plant or herb, I look at the way the plant grows, I examine its smell and study its shape, and sometimes this reveals its possible medicinal use. If at all possible, particularly with varieties of herbs and plants previously unknown to me, I like to see and study them in their natural habitat.

One day when I was at work in our main clinic, Auchenkyle, in the south-west of Scotland, I took a brief stroll at lunch-time. Surrounding this clinic are some 20 acres of unspoilt woodland, untouched by chemicals or fertilisers, where we have an impressive organic nursery. As I wandered along, a chestnut fell out of a tree, onto my head. It hurt, but not for long. When the chestnut hit the ground the rough shell burst open displaying a beautiful shiny nut.

I picked it up and could not help wondering what message this shiny fruit had for me. I was aware that the horse chestnut has long been known as a good remedy for blood circulatory problems such as haemorrhoids and varicose veins, but there was nothing in this chestnut to indicate a similarity to the circulatory system, and I wondered if there was a hidden message that I had failed to interpret. On closer inspection I imagined that I recognised the shape of a foetus and I then thought of the circulatory problems of pregnant women, and I decided to show the chestnut to a few midwives. Like me, most of them failed to identify the message, and several were not impressed by my train of thought. One midwife, however, recognised the possible meaning. She agreed that, with a little imagination, this indeed reminded her of the foetus of a baby.

I knew that the chestnut was an effective treatment for varicose veins and haemorrhoids, and I decided to use the chestnut extract – Aesculus Hippocastanum – for women who had difficulties in becoming pregnant. I tried this with a number of my patients and the success rate was certainly encouraging. I then decided to use the chestnut extract for women who were approaching their delivery date, and I asked them to take ten drops twice daily during the final six weeks prior to delivery. The results were even more encouraging because a considerable number of them told me that they had a very much easier delivery than previously experienced. The message was very clear to me. Scientifically, this may not be considered a valid exercise, but I had learned about the purpose of the horse chestnut, although its properties only became obvious once I had studied and tested it. Results cannot be disputed, so I was delighted to see the successful results of this particular herbal remedy, before, during and after pregnancy. I had asked a number of midwives to help me in this study and they spoke of their appreciation, and the remedy Aesculaforce, combining the horse chestnut extract with some other ingredients, has become a well-known remedy which has been of great help to many.

The medical profession is often critical and adverse to the use of herbs because there is little or no proof or scientific data available to ensure its safety and effectiveness. However, it is an old and established science. Herbal remedies have been used for centuries, in fact, as long as mankind has populated this earth. Dr Vogel, now well into his nineties, has written in depth on herbs, roots, plants and flowers, and his book *The Nature Doctor* can be found in many households worldwide where it is frequently used as a reference book. He has recognised, for example, that during pregnancy and afterwards the mother is often troubled by phlebitis, inflammation of the veins, thrombosis and perhaps embolism, and his advice is to use remedies such as Hyperisan and St John's Wort.

Named after the apostle, this is another herb with an apt name. The plant's little leaves are dotted with tiny holes, hence the Latin name *hypericum perforatum*. The small leaves seem to encourage touching and stroking, and this plant is the basis of Dr Vogel's St John's Wort Oil – the healing balm for many apparently unrelated problems. Used externally, this oil gives a soothing effect and helps with circulation. As a tincture, it can be used internally – ten drops twice a day. St John's Wort, with its healing characteristics, is greatly beneficial to pregnant women or new mothers who are experiencing circulatory problems, varicose veins or haemorrhoids.

The yarrow plant and arnica are both equally important in herbal medicine. The same goes for pulsatilla, which is used as a remedy to regulate the circulation. This remedy, however, should only be taken during pregnancy in a low homoeopathic potency. The stinging nettle, which provides an injection of blood-cleansing properties, is a true gift of nature.

If a nursing mother is afraid that she may not have enough milk to feed the infant, she would be wise to use a remedy containing urtica extract or the remedy Urticalcin – three to five tablets, twice a day – to overcome calcium or silicea deficiency. Such a deficiency frequently occurs after the birth of a baby, and this remedy is a useful preventative, especially if the mother were to develop signs of glandular problems. A lack of calcium during pregnancy might create an inherent deficiency, because the foetus needs, and takes, a formidable amount of calcium from the mother and, if she does not get enough of this in her diet, Urticalcin can be a valuable ally.

Silicea is also necessary and can be obtained from sauerkraut, horsetail and the hemp nettle. Silicea intake is twice as effective if taken together with a calcium preparation. There is an excellent tonic, which can be used before and after the baby's birth, called Vitaforce which will supply the body with extra strength.

Herbs for Pregnancy, written by Ann McIntyre, contains some very useful information on herbs that are safe to use during pregnancy. Since the dawning of consciousness nothing has been more revered than the miracle of birth, and science has made great advances towards making the expectant mother as safe as possible. How can she take more care of herself, than through watching the food she eats and the herbs she uses, both provided by nature. Alfalfa, watercress, parsley, and rosehips are wonderful remedies when used as a general tonic. For morning-sickness, remember that raspberry-leaf tea, spearmint tea or, in the case of digestive problems, peppermint tea, papaya tablets or charcoal tablets are tried and tested remedies.

For sleeplessness expectant mothers can safely take remedies containing valeriana, such as Dormeasan from Dr Vogel – 20 drops before going to bed, or Melissa (lemon balm), Avena sativa (oat extract), Passiflora (the passion flower), Humulus (hops), and Lupulinum (hop grains). All are excellent herbal remedies for insomnia. I can remember the days when the merest mention of raspberry tea would bring a smile to people's faces, but in latter years it has become widely accepted as an excellent aid to an easier birth. It is very important that a pregnant mother drinks the right beverages and I often advise that coffee be replaced by a very palatable substitute called 'Bambu coffee' which contains a number of healthy ingredients. Herbal teas are also becoming more popular. So much can be done to help us lead a much happier and healthier existence. For example, to help the hair and the skin and to strengthen the nails, take three to five Urticalcin tablets, twice daily. Kidney functions are enhanced by taking golden grass tea.

Now to pregnancy-related problems of a different kind. Stretch marks can be minimised or avoided by Calendula or using Calendula ointment. A nervous disposition can be relieved by Avena sativa – ten drops twice daily and sore nipples will improve if you use Golden Seal or PauPau extract or ointment. Sometimes help can be so easily obtained, for example, to improve the milk production nursing mothers are advised to drink a concoction of honey with the juices of green vegetables, such as parsley, lettuce, spinach or celery, three or four times a day. Aniseed oil is also helpful in these situations.

During pregnancy one should always be very careful with medicines; therefore, minute homoeopathic doses are often best, because certain herbal preparations can be rather potent and in some cases could even stimulate contractions. As with all medicines, however, you should always check with your doctor, herbal practitioner, midwife or health visitor.

I very often prescribe Ignatia or Echinaforce. Not only is this remedy very helpful for the immune system, but also for minor problems when a natural antibiotic is required. For everyday problems, such as a common cold, diarrhoea, minor infections, or whenever an antibiotic would be prescribed, this remedy is of tremendous value. Tests at the University of Munich have underlined the benefits of this remedy and I have great admiration for my mentor and tutor, Dr Alfred Vogel, who has worked so much with echinacea that his remedy Echinaforce has become my most reliable ally in the treatments I prescribe to many of my patients. Many years ago, Dr Vogel worked with the Sioux Indians in North America, where he learned how they used this plant. He then studied its properties and realised its importance to the immune system. The plant's characteristics can be easily tested by arranging a bunch of these flowers in a vase and deliberately forgetting to replenish the water. It is remarkable how long they will survive and this is indicative of the effect it has when taken as a herbal preparation. No sooner is this remedy taken than it immediately stimulates an increase in the number of white blood-cells. Use of this remedy will rapidly prevent the formation of the enzyme hyaluronidase, therefore, infections cannot spread. Furthermore, echinacea has a stimulating effect on the lymph system.

To my mind Echinaforce is one of the most versatile remedies available and I could not imagine what it would be like if I were not able to prescribe this to my patients. If you have read my book *Home and Herbal Remedies* you will not be surprised at my enthusiasm for this plant, because I have supplied many examples where this plant has provided the solution where other, more drastic, conventional medicines have failed. I have often prescribed Echinaforce for pregnant women and young babies. Not so long ago, a patient phoned me for advice because her baby had constant diarrhoea. Everything had been tried and I advised that the young child should be given a few drops of Echinaforce every day and, indeed, she phoned me later to let me know that this had solved the problem.

This reminds me of a school friend who studied medicine and married one of his fellow students, also a doctor. One day they arrived on my doorstep in Scotland. They were happy in their marriage which was obvious to anyone who came in contact with them. I was delighted to see them, but sad when I learned of their visit's ulterior motive. Apart from coming to see me for old time's sake, they also came seeking advice. They were desperate to have a family but so far nothing had come of it. I gave them some advice, which I will describe in a later chapter on the subject of infertility, and four months later they phoned to tell me that she was pregnant. Eventually, I was informed that they had become the proud parents of a beautiful and much loved baby girl.

Six weeks later I received another phone call from my friend. He was most upset and told me that the baby was desperately ill and that they were afraid they might lose her. They did not know what was wrong, but the baby had continuous diarrhoea and was in severe danger of dehydration. All kinds of antibiotics had been tried, but to no avail. I was very anxious for them, but at the same time I was also very annoyed because I had told them numerous times about the remedial properties of Echinacea and yet, in the fight for his daughter's life, he had forgotten all about it. I told him to give the baby a few drops of Echinaforce immediately. Within a week he phoned to say that the baby was on the mend and today this same baby is now a doctor and I know that her parents have told her that her life was saved by a simple herbal remedy.

This took place a long time ago, but it is only one of many case histories I have collected on this one remedy. Many pregnant women have also benefited from this remedy, and it should be remembered that most conditions are sparked off by an apparently innocent ailment, a common cold for instance. I would not like to be accused of encouraging people to become hypochondriacs, but it is important to remember that many conditions are allowed to develop because the early warning signs are ignored. Maybe they will disappear eventually, but I for one would not like to take this for granted. It should be remembered that women are at their most vulnerable during pregnancy and it is so important that the right measures are taken to avoid the development of a more serious condition. It is wonderful to realise that nature is our best friend, and never is this more obvious than when we look at a newborn baby and see the perfection of life. What could be better than to use God's gift of nature to alleviate human suffering.

I considered myself very fortunate when I succeeded in buying the oldest herbal pharmacy in Scotland. This pharmacy dates back more than a century, and I was most intrigued by the documents I found in the cellar, going back to the days when, for the common people, especially if they lived in rural areas, a doctor's assistance was near enough impossible. In those days there were no midwives or health visitors with medical training and back-up. Most treatments were handed down from mother to daughter, mostly by word of mouth, and it is these proven methods that have so often been ridiculed in recent years. What I was most interested in, especially with regard to this present book, was what was then considered effective and safe for use before, during and after pregnancy. I was amazed at how many of the herbal remedies mentioned in this chapter were in use in those days. It was fascinating to read about the attention paid to minor complaints which today we would often ignore. For example, I am increasingly worried that babies are often present in the same room where the family sit smoking and watching television. The noise and smoke are not conducive to a baby's health; rays from a television screen adversely affect the immune system of both adults and babies. I am increasingly worried when I see babies spend their days indoors, too often in rooms which are artificially lit. It is important babies get plenty of fresh air and are harmonised – this is particularly important for young babies.

In the pharmacy I mentioned, I found a small booklet written by a herbalist, who counted the Rt Hon W.E. Gladstone among his patients. In an extract of a speech made at Guy's Hospital in London on 26 March 1890, it was mentioned that the origin of the medical profession could be traced back to two sources. One of these, the observation of nature, produced the herbalist. Gladstone was not aware at the time that botany would, in later years, be considered as a recognised branch of medical education. Botany, in itself, is a beautiful and interesting subject to study, exercising the mind without fatiguing it and stimulating the imagination without leading it astray. Instead, it trains us to carefully observe nature, noticing the remarkably powerful healing qualities of plants. In his speech, published on 27 March 1890 in the *Daily News*, Gladstone told a little anecdote which, simple though it was, still illustrated what he meant. He related an instance where he had been given the task of cutting wood. By sheer accident one day he cut his finger on the sharp edge of the axe and drew blood. He realised that he had no pocket handkerchief and so he found a leaf which he placed on the cut to staunch the bleeding. He told his audience that he was honour-bound to say that it was not the result of botanical knowledge, but merely an impulse. But the curious result was that the healing of this cut took only half the time it would have taken without the assistance of nature. He could not help but think that there were great treasures in nature, more than had been explored or suspected.

Botanists believe that there is scarcely a plant that grows which, on being analysed, will not be found to contain certain medicinal properties. Although I should be used to it by now, it never ceases to amaze me how beneficial plants, herbs, leaves and roots can be to specific medical conditions. With great interest I read every word in the book *Valuable Herbal Prescriptions*, and I was intrigued to see a section on spectacles and children. It should be remembered that this book dates from the days of candles and gaslighting, which were very much softer than the artificial light we use today. An elderly person who remembers the days of candle-light will also remember that they seldom saw a child or youth wearing spectacles. I know that it is a controversial statement, but I am afraid that many cases of impaired vision in children nowadays can be attributed principally to thoughtlessness. From the book I quote:

The mother dills baby in her lap and allows it to gaze to its heart's content at the gaslight, crooning to it. The mother who can afford a basinette takes particular care to line the basinette and the interior of the hood with pure white. Little bapsy, whichever way it looks, has its eyes fixed on about the last thing capable of resting its sight. And there is also that little white cot; when you have that little white cot fixed up with white wood and white curtain, be kind enough for the baby's sake to fix the cot with the gaslight behind it and allow me now to inform you that the two best shades for the lining of the cot or basinette are black or dark green, and if you do not want to see your baby sooner or later wearing spectacles, you will do well to remember this. Let your final instructions to nurse be that when she reaches the park with that nice novelette, to take particular care to keep the child's back to the sun. Babies are attracted by the sun or gaslight and either can pave the way for mischief to their sight.

I have quoted this section from this old English book because I was touched to read that so much consideration was given to the eyesight of small babies. Today, it is far from unusual for young children to need spectacles. Not only that, but I am increasingly worried by the variety of eyesight problems we come across at relatively young ages. It might be going a bit far to line the cot with black or dark green material, but as for artificial light, I am quite sure that insufficient consideration is given to the baby's needs, through sheer thoughtlessness.

The book also specifies that chamomile water should be used to cleanse matter from the baby's eyes. Thankfully, there are still a considerable number of mothers who use chamomile when cleaning their baby's eyes. Indeed, many of the hundreds of recipes and recommendations found in the cellars of Napier's Pharmacy in Edinburgh, dating back to the nineteenth century, are still in use in the latter part of the twentieth century. Many of these old remedies have stood the test of time.

When I visit other countries I always go out of my way to find out what kind of remedies were used, especially if no medical help is, or was, available. I am very pleased that herbal medicine is once again getting well-deserved recognition and is no longer regarded as an old-fashioned and outdated form of medicine. It is far from that. Always remember that God's promise to mankind was that we will be given food to exist and herbs for healing.

6

Acupuncture

A highly-strung lady had made an appointment to see me at the clinic and it took me a while to break the ice and gain her confidence. She was pregnant with her first child and she admitted that she was scared witless and did not know how she was going to cope with the delivery. We discussed the physical part of giving birth and she accusingly countered that by saying that I could only speak as a spectator, and that my knowledge was gained from books. Of course, I had never been through the process myself, but I did tell her that my wife had given birth to four children, that I had grandchildren and also that many patients had told me about their experiences. Sometimes these stories are tales of woe, but generally it is seen as an outstandingly happy experience, There was, I felt, no need for her to worry. For the time being I advised her on relaxation methods and remedies and, at a later appointment, she brought her husband with her who seemed even more uptight then his wife. We had quite a chat and they made me promise that she could count on me for support during her pregnancy.

At her next visit to the clinic she was very enthusiastic and happy and she told me that, because I was a qualified acupuncturist, she was hoping I would agree to be at her bedside when her time came and help her during labour with the aid of acupuncture. Unfortunately, I had to tell her that because of my commitments in various clinics I could not promise to be there, as I would not know where I would be and might even be out of the country when she went into labour. Therefore, it would be unfair to promise that I would be there in person. She began to cry and admitted that she had clung to this as her only hope. I sympathised with her and promised that I would do my very best to be around when she was due. I promised that when her time came and if I was in the area, I would be present.

It was a wonderful birth. Acupuncture has been used for many centuries and is extremely effective in times of need when it can be applied as a means of anaesthesia. I admit that it is time-consuming and because of my commitments I cannot usually make myself freely available, but this birth was an excellent reminder of just how effective this treatment can be.

Acupuncture anaesthesia is not very widely used in the West, but I had administered this on a number of occasions, especially during my years in the Far East. When I initially studied acupuncture in Germany I never even considered that eventually this study would take me to China, where acupuncture is used a great deal as a local anaesthetic. There, I also became familiar with the therapy called moxabustion, which is based on the principle of acupuncture. A qualified acupuncturist, who decides to help a mother who is scared to go through the birth process unaided, can be of great assistance.

During pregnancy many encephalins and endorphins are released by the mother's body, and while the baby is making its way into the world these natural morphines will help to control the pain and support the mother. There is no problem with receiving acupuncture treatment during pregnancy, although it is generally advisable to avoid this during the first and final three months. In the early months there is a small risk that acupuncture could cause an abortion, while during the latter months it could possibly induce a premature birth. The chances of this happening are small, but are, nevertheless, better avoided. This should always be explained whenever women seek acupuncture treatment and any worthwhile practitioner will ask if there is any indication of a pregnancy.

I began using acupuncture in my Scottish clinic some 25 years ago, and at the time there was very considerable opposition to this form of therapy. Today, however, it is viewed in a very different light. I remember that when I lectured in medical establishments in those early days I was often criticised for introducing these new methods. Actually, this made little sense because acupuncture is one of the oldest forms of medicine in the world, as it has been practised in China for some 6,000 years. It is a wonderful form of treatment as many of my patients will testify. During pregnancy, back troubles are rather common and here again, acupuncture can bring about enormous relief.

The traditional method of acupuncture is safer and more effective during pregnancy than the modern version which is widely referred to as electro-acupuncture. Until recently acupuncture used to be referred to as 'fringe medicine', yet it has recently caught the attention of many physicians and practitioners. Unfortunately, there are people who think that they will be able to learn this science during a few weekend seminars and go on to join the list of qualified practitioners. This adversely affects the reputation of capable and qualified acupuncturists who are so often unfairly referred to as 'charlatans'. It is important to point out that it takes years of learning and experience to become a capable acupuncturist. Despite all the studies I have undertaken and the many, many years of experience I have had, I still study all the new forms as they are introduced. It is a poor acupuncturist who does not understand and study its philosophy to the full for it is this philosophy of acupuncture which is so important. It tells us how to restore harmony in the body when, for whatever reason this has become unbalanced, how to use the needles, not only according to what is written in the book, but also intuitively; feeling what would be most suitable for the patient.

More research papers have been published on the subject of acupuncture than on any other single topic in medicine over recent years and while these have been very helpful, it is experience that counts. I have come across many problems with so-called acupuncturists who lack the feeling for what this treatment is all about. It was not until I studied in China that I came to appreciate fully the philosophy behind this science. Not only does one need to be a very good diagnostician, one needs to know where and how to look for the pulses. Today, acupuncture is probably the most widely recognised of all alternative treatment methods. I know that latterly many hospitals have decided to include this form of therapy in their curriculum. I have often been invited to speak to and advise allopathic practitioners and I have been happy to do so, as I have also been happy to assist with acupuncture treatment during pregnancies or deliveries.

Despite the abundance of scientific data published on the subject of acupuncture, something is often overlooked. Acupuncture practice is not something that has evolved from modern scientific studies; it is an art that is founded on a philosophy and on principles that go back some five or six thousand years. One of my most impressive teachers, Prof. Tsjang, always maintained that acupuncture is only as good as the practitioner. It requires a lot of understanding, careful handling, thought and patience.

It is impossible to explain in a nutshell how acupuncture really works. Although I have practised this art for more than 30 years now, it still surprises me. Indeed, I prefer to call it an art and often, when I see a good acupuncturist at work, I look on him more as an artist than as a doctor. The effects created by the needles are both subjective and objective. The peculiar sensation that the patients feel after the needles are placed and activated is called 'chi' in Chinese. It is mostly experienced as a strange, but not uncomfortable feeling. For acupuncture anaesthesia to be successful it is essential that adequate chi is encouraged.

When I worked in a hospital in Sri Lanka we were taught the six different effects of acupuncture:

- It is most widely recognised as an analgesic pain-relieving technique, which works by raising the pain threshold. This is the psychological base of acupuncture anaesthesia and explains similarly produced acupuncture analgesia during therapy. Some acupuncture points can be more or less effective, depending on the patient.
- The needle placement and the use of specific acupuncture points results in sedation which explains why sometimes a patient may fall asleep during treatment and wake up very much refreshed.
- Also very important is the homoeostatic or regulatory effect, which means there is an adjustment of the internal environment of the body towards a better balance. The fourteen meridians the body has in the yin and yang system (yin and yang means negative and positive) carry hundreds of points and it is vital that the right points are chosen and that the practitioner is well-taught and competent so that he knows what he is doing. The balance between the sympathetic and the para-sympathetic system of the autonomic nervous system and the endocrine system plays a very large role.
- There is the immune enhancing action of acupuncture whereby the body's resistance is realigned. This has been known to produce an increase in the white corpuscles or leucocytes, antibodies, gammaglobulins and other substances which increase resistance in the body, which explains why acupuncture is also helpful in the case of infections.
- A further important factor in acupuncture is that it speeds up the motor recovery in a patient who may have become paralysed. Although this paralysis may only be temporary, it responds well to acupuncture treatment. The explanation, although very complex, is the antidromic stimulation and the reactivation through a biofeedback mechanism operating through the different cells of the spinal chord.

- The last objective effect in the list is the psychological effect. Acupuncture has a calming and tranquillising action, different to mere sedation. This is the reason why acupuncture is so helpful during childbirth. It is believed to be due to an action on the mid-brain reticular formation, and certain other parts of the brain. It has also been known to have an effect on the metabolic chemistry and the brain tissue. This particular effect has nothing whatsoever to do with hypnosis or auto-suggestion. These effects are the result of acupuncture and are therefore not a pre-condition of its success. It really has nothing to do with hypnotism, autogenic training or auto-suggestion. The automatic nervous system is also believed to play an important role in acupuncture and there is experimental evidence that suggests that along the sympathetic plexuses surrounding blood vessels, some of the acupuncture impulses have travelled between the spinal cord and the brain.

I once attended a lecture given by Dr Bruce Pomeranz, Professor at the Neuro-Biology Unit at Toronto University, who suggested that naturally occurring endorphins play a prominent part in acupuncture. He believed that they bind onto the opiate receptors in the brain cells, and with the endorphins, released by acupuncture, could produce an analgesic effect.

Research in China has shown that endorphins originate in the pituitary gland and encephalins in the mid-brain. The pituitary endorphins are secreted as part of a long chain molecule called beta-lipotropin. The mechanism of how encephalins inhibit pain may be indirect – instead of acting directly on the receiving nerve cell, it is known that the substance may block the release of acting neuro-transmitters, such as acetyl choline and glutomate, thereby reducing the receiving cells' excitatory input. At the moment, clinical trials are being conducted in association with Prof. Pomeranz in order to determine whether in acupuncture anaesthesia and in childbirth the effect of acupuncture to relieve pain may be potentiated using the antipeptidasis. These findings have been confirmed and I have been amazed how well this has worked in childbirth.

There is much one can do without a practitioner at your side and at their request I have instructed a number of pregnant women on how to use certain energy points during the birth process. My book, *Body Energy*, discusses a great number of these points and describes how they can be used by the individual to relieve pain. We call this acupressure, a useful do-it-yourself technique that is quite easy and also totally safe.

The body is not only electrical in nature, but also has its positive and negative poles. The heart represents the negative side, while the brain (the right side) represents the positive. There should be a balance. Contact healing is a method of contacting the electrical sensors in the body and acupressure treats those various points of the body which relate to the different areas, glands and organs. There are a great number of publications on acupressure, most with very useful advice. Always remember that it cannot do any harm, it is simple to apply and it does not cost a penny. I have had numerous letters from grateful patients who have read *Body Energy* and have applied what they thought most suitable to their particular circumstances.

One comparatively new way of treating pain is by way of a small machine which the patient can safely use at home, called TENS – Transcutaneous Electrical Nerve Stimulations. I now know a number of people who have this equipment at home. Many mothers have told me how much help this little machine has been during the birth of their baby. This application of electrical stimulations on the nerve system for the relief of acute or chronic pain is of a non-invasive nature and the user-friendliness of this machine, initially under medical supervision, makes it an attractive form of pain relief.

Prof. Wall of the University College, London, and Prof. Melzack of Canada have worked together on research into pain and their findings and those of other researchers confirm conclusively that the application of electrodes to external points of pain can achieve a worthwhile rate of success. The psychological mechanism of TENS and its techniques in electro-therapy are based on the theories of acupuncture and indeed application of the electrodes to the relevant acupuncture points has been found to be very effective. TENS as a technique is becoming increasingly popular in pain-relieving clinics throughout the world, particularly when used in conjunction with other forms of remedial therapy. It is advisable that this type of apparatus be used under the direction of a practitioner who can recommend the frequency of the treatment and the placement points for the patches. As a general guideline it is usually necessary to have one 30-minute session daily. It should be noted that, although the TENS machine must not be used during pregnancy, it is of great help during childbirth.

7

Cranial Osteopathy

Occasionally, when I have some spare time, I accompany my wife to the Open Air Museum where she is a guide. This museum is part of the Holy Land Foundation in the west of the Netherlands and aims to explain and show the visitor how the Egyptians, Jews, Greeks and Romans lived in biblical times. It is very interesting to meet the public and get involved in some of the discussions that develop. Earlier this year I met a young couple there and I noticed that the father was carrying a young baby. When I looked at the baby I immediately noticed that there was something wrong with the baby's hands and feet. During our conversation I learned that this baby had been handicapped since birth. Apparently, it had been a very difficult birth and I discovered that the baby might be handicapped because the mother had been under medication during pregnancy. Unfortunately, all the medical specialists had reached the same conclusion that this baby would never be able to use his hands or feet.

When I hear stories like this my heart bleeds, because I always feel that everything possible should be done to prevent such problems. I have seen too many babies with medical conditions caused at birth, often resulting from Caesarean section or forceps delivery, and the best advice I can give these parents is to try cranial osteopathy with the help of a qualified practitioner in this field.

Cranial osteopathy is a specific science and is best summed up by the Duchess of Newcastle's saying, 'Motion is the life of all things.' Some beliefs in medical history have been around so long that no one has ever considered doubting them. Long ago it was concluded that the fontanelle – the soft boneless area in the skull of a baby – grows slowly together into one hard, bony area, the skull or cranium, so that the bones form an enclosure for the brain. There never seemed to be a reason to doubt this fact even though one does not see or feel the cranium moving. However, this changed in the early seventies.

During an operation the American, John E. Upledger, noticed movement in the cerebral membrane or the meninges. During tests he discovered that the cranial bones also moved, which intrigued him and he decided to investigate further. On the basis of his research Dr Upledger developed a treatment method for a variety of painful conditions, such as back pain or migraine, and also for co-ordination problems, learning and behavioural problems, emotional disturbances and post-trauma conditions. The rhythmic movement of the cranial bones, the so-called cranial-sacral rhythm, became the starting-point of cranial osteopathic treatment. The name cranial-sacral therapy came about because of the bones that, together with the vertebrae, enclose the central nervous system. The cranial bones, a combination of the frontal or coronal bone and the temporal bone, is known as the cranium. The sacrum is the Latin name for the bone located immediately above the coccyx or the tail-bone.

The brains and the spinal marrow are covered by three membranes protecting a circulating fluid. The outer meninges or membrane is called the *dura mater*, and covers the inside of the cranium. This membrane is connected to the inside of the cranium and also to a few areas of the spinal column. The membrane ensures that the fluid cannot escape. Brain and spinal fluid is produced and regulated by a mechanism in the brain, and because the mass of fluid occasionally increases or decreases, the pressure applied by the fluid to the membrane is variable. It is this variance that is called the cranial-sacral rhythm.

Scientific research has determined that the seams between the cranial bones contain blood vessels, nerves and connective tissue. This structural design allows movement of the cranial bones along with the cranial membrane. When the cranial-sacral rhythm had been recognised, Dr Upledger investigated the frequency of movement of the cranium and it is thought that the mass of brain and spinal fluid changes from six to 12 times each minute, causing a fluctuating pressure on the cranial membrane and bones.

The cranial-sacral system may be compared to a hydraulic system. This means that the pressure applied at a certain point is spontaneously applied throughout the system. Imagine a balloon filled with water. When pressure is applied at one point, movement at another point is noticeable. In this manner every movement within the system affects the overall system. Because the cranial-sacral system surrounds the brains and the spinal fluid, it influences the performance of important body functions. It is generally known that the brains and the bone marrow co-ordinate our observations and movements. Perhaps it is less well-known that other body functions are also affected, such as breathing, digestion and the heart beat. The pituitary gland is located in the brain and this gland determines and regulates the function of other glands such as the thyroid, the adrenals and the ovaries.

Disturbance of the cranial-sacral rhythm and blockage of the movement of the membranes and the cranium will have a detrimental effect on the brains and the bone marrow, causing an impediment to certain body functions. Such a disturbance can be brought about by a physical trauma such as an accident, a viral infection, poisoning or a surgical operation. What happens is that too much pressure is applied to the cranial membrane, obstructing movement of the cranial bones.

The aim of cranial-sacral therapy is to remove the blockages within the cranial-sacral system, allowing the cranial membrane and bones to move without restrictions, and recover their natural rhythm. In order to understand the actual treatment, one should visualise the cranial bones as horny handles of the cranial membrane. By using them as a sort of handle it is possible to influence the cranial-sacral system.

An experienced therapist or practitioner can observe the cranial-sacral rhythm with his or her hands in nearly every part of the body. This allows certain areas to be localised where malfunctioning is diagnosed, by a restriction in mobility. The treatment is aimed at investigating and improving the movement of the rhythm in various parts of the system. In order to do this it is not necessary to apply heavy pressure anywhere, as a light touch is more than sufficient. When this corrective movement has been applied the body will call upon its own correction mechanism and the healing process can start to bring the system back into balance.

Scientific research in 1975, at the American Michigan State University, gave Dr Upledger the opportunity to conclusively prove the existence of the cranial-sacral system. Healthcare institutes in the USA now make wide use of this knowledge and many people receive cranial osteopathic treatment. John Upledger was one of the first to be involved in scientific research in this area, although movement of the cranium had already been observed by other practitioners. I feel privileged to have had the opportunity to attend several seminars given by William G. Sutherland, who was a highly trained and capable osteopath. His lectures dealt with the purpose of movement and I still have all my notes from these lectures, which have been of great help to me in my treatment of patients.

Sutherland explained that in his early research he practised upon himself with the aid of a specially designed helmet to which a number of thumbscrews had been attached. By turning these screws he practised his theories by applying a variable pressure to different parts of the scalp, thus deliberately blocking normal movement. According to Sutherland's wife, she observed noticeable behavioural changes as a result of these experiments. Sutherland also discovered that by causing an obstruction of certain movements of the cranium, not only could he bring on headaches and migraines, but also some of his physical movements became laboured and he experienced disturbances in some of his organs. He successfully used this knowledge in the treatment of his patients. He was, in many ways, ahead of his time so the necessary technology was not in place in the first half of this century to make his findings available to the rest of the medical community. To my mind, however, Sutherland was the real inventor of what is now termed cranial osteopathy.

Osteopathy, although an old form of treatment, is no more than a modern scientific development of the two oldest treatment forms known to man: massage and manipulation. It is, in essence, a natural therapy which seeks to overcome a wide range of diseases, disabilities and pains, which result from disturbances of the body's framework and moving parts. Just as structural engineers undergo lengthy training to help them to understand the mechanics of bridges, dams and highrise buildings, so osteopaths follow an extensive study including anatomy, physiology and pathology of the human body, to equip them with the necessary knowledge to analyse problems and diagnose complaints using a variety of clinical skills backed up by necessary X-ray examinations and bio-chemical tests. The treatment, designed to correct the faults revealed by a thorough medical investigation, is gentle and rarely causes discomfort. In most cases it is followed by explanation and advice to help prevent a recurrence of the problem. If other treatment is required, the osteopath will immediately refer the patient to the appropriate source of help.

I have been very fortunate in my teachers, one of whom was Dr Len Allan, a student of Sutherland's, who taught me a great deal about cranial osteopathy. I was also taught by the American, George Ivan Carter, whose work I have described in *Body Energy*. I remember that when he was quite elderly, he handed me an old press article, dated 1949, describing some of his work. It said that

American doctors did not know what was happening in the human body and that the American people were getting more and more unhealthy year by year, but that through the simple system designed by George Ivan Carter, a large number of people had been fortunate and enjoyed much better health. This system was called 'Body Symmetry' and Carter's system, clearly derived from osteopathy, became so widely known and praised that the medical profession had little option but to recognise it.

According to Carter, when Newton discovered the law of gravity, he missed something very important; that gravity is responsible for man's ills. Right from the embryo stage, gravity pulls man's entire physical structure out of balance. What happens to the head is of utmost importance because it holds the brain and all those nerve paths. In all my life I have not seen one perfectly balanced skull. In fact, I dare say, that there is not one bone in the body that is correctly balanced. Most of the skulls I see have mastoid bones out of place, or one side of the head is lower than the other. It's no wonder that the owner does not feel very well. The mastoid bone is the springboard to health.

I have studied Carter at work – aligning those out of place bones and using the first form of cranial osteopathy – and one could not fail to recognise his skill. He claims that it takes about 500 movements, just to start getting the body into balance. He then carefully squeezes the patient's head as if it were a piece of fruit. For the duration of the treatment he would work with a very high degree of concentration. In his time he had a success rate of over 80 per cent. I remember asking him about retarded children and children who were slightly injured during Caesarean or forceps delivery and, at that time, Carter said that America's seven million retarded children could benefit from this particular therapy. More important, said Carter, was that a large percentage of retarded children could benefit to such an extent that most would be able to lead a perfectly normal life. I am not sure that that statement was entirely correct, because he may have been over-enthusiastic, but I do know that much can be done if a baby has suffered an injury at birth. One of my more recent teachers, Denis Brooks, became known for his saying, 'Find it, fix it and leave it'. His book, *Cranial Osteopathy*, has been of great guidance to me in my work. He refers to the remarkable works of Dr Charlotte Weaver and Dr Naylor, printed in 1936–37, which opened the floodgates to an understanding of the cranial structures and their characteristics. Dr Weaver and Dr Naylor, and later Dr Melvyn Page, all studied the interaction between calcium and phosphorus in a balanced form within the human body which are both essential for the endocrine glands' interplay. The results of their work suggested some new approaches to some cranial problems and also re-affirmed the need to balance the sympathetic and parasympathetic nervous system.

Ronald R. McCatty was another pupil of Denis Brooks. I have known him for many years and his book on cranial osteopathy, *Essentials of Craniosacral Osteopathy*, contains valuable advice for other practitioners. He, too, thought highly of Denis Brooks as a cranial osteopath and suggested some interesting approaches. I have watched him at work many times and it was always impressive when he used very gentle manipulative treatment to adjust certain conditions. When a baby is born, the moulding which takes place during the birth, will decide the shape and bone structure of the head. A Caesarean section or a forceps delivery can affect the cranial setting of a baby. The anaesthetic the mother receives can also contribute to a delayed birth and I think it is a shame if a forceps delivery becomes necessary. If performed by an experienced doctor or midwife, however, it can be to the baby's benefit because prolonged labour and the accompanying stress may be avoided.

Birth injuries are usually recognisable as slight bruising to the skin. With each generation it would appear that generally the foetus is, at the birth, too large for the birth canal. The main cause of undue distortion of the membrane and cartilage of the infant's skull is usually from either induced birth or forceps delivery. Lately it has been suggested that post-natal depression, backache and pelvic disturbances may also be caused by a forced birth.

Most people believe that time heals all, but these conditions can become serious in later life. This can even lead to permanent disability and that is why I consider the work of a cranial osteopath to be so important. The frontal bone covers the behavioural centres of the cerebrum and this can easily be affected by a forced or unnatural birth. Neglect of this damage can cause disturbances in infancy and may continue into adult life.

So far, I have only mentioned the cranial-sacral system, but it goes without saying that any impairment of the nervous system can also have severe consequences. Cranial osteopathy is a reliable and safe treatment method for these conditions and, in the treatment of babies or infants, a gentleness of touch is particularly necessary and should only be carried out by very skilled hands. Cranial base decompression may be attempted only by a very knowledgeable and experienced practitioner, who has studied his subject thoroughly. I also would like to suggest that women who become pregnant with their first child during their thirties and forties, often find it helpful to consult a cranial osteopath as soon as they know they are pregnant for a check-up, so that possible problems during their pregnancy or at the birth may be avoided.

The sacrum is suspended between the ilia by strong bands and varies considerably in shape, size and volume. It got its name because of its close association with the new life created during pregnancy within the pelvic bowl and indeed, it forms the posterior wall of that cavity. The female sacrum and pelvis tends to be shorter and broader than the male, but the vestigial articular tubercles are more prominent and larger in men. This has been particularly relevant to many of the misalignments I have been asked to treat in women after they have given birth. If the pelvis is out of place or misaligned, it can lead to serious problems later on. It, therefore, would make sense if women were to consult a qualified osteopath for a check-up six weeks after the birth of their baby.

There is much more that can be said on the subject of cranial osteopathy, but I have deliberately tried to restrict it to those circumstances pertinent to the subject of this book. I should also mention the Fallopian tubes and the ovaries. Tender or swollen ovaries could indicate an ovarian tumour, fibroids or inflammation. This need not be serious, but an enlarged ovary could indicate an imminent period when ovulation occurs, or the early stages of pregnancy. Usually those fibroids are hard and consist of solid matter. The Fallopian tubes, which are the funnel at the end of the ovaries, can easily become blocked, and, when swollen and sensitive, require urgent medical attention because this can be an indication of an ectopic pregnancy. Petasites – ten drops three times a day before meals – will be helpful in such cases. Genetic deficiencies can never be ruled out. Sudden shock or trauma resulting in pelvic lesions from a cerebral spinal fluid interruption can cause major problems.

Fortunately, in most cases, everything goes well. If, however, there are problems for whatever reasons, or expectant mothers have had problems during previous pregnancies or births, consult your doctor or practitioner. These newer fields of medicine are mostly based on common sense, although as you well know, these therapies are not new, but as old as mankind itself. Do not take 'no' for an answer, because over the years I have seen so many benefits from cranial osteopathy.

As Paracelsus, the German-Swiss philosopher, said, 'If a new idea can be fitted into the authoritarian brainwork, we are apt to accept it uncritically, whereas if it breaks new ground we are likely to reject it.'

8

New Arrival

Hooray . . . Hooray . . . the baby has arrived. What happiness for the mother, the father, brothers and sisters, family, neighbours and friends. Lots of flowers and presents and joy at the arrival of the newborn. Mostly, mothers feel relieved and wonder afterwards why they worried about it in the first place. This little creature lying peacefully beside them is a perfect example of what nature is all about. Yet, sometimes one should not completely rule out problems later on.

I was thinking recently about a young couple who were so worried when it was suspected that she was pregnant, because they had only just set up home and felt that, financially, they were not in a position to make a commitment to the future. At the same time they realised that this was truly a happy occasion, if only the price wasn't so high. They had not long been married and there was still so much they had planned to do before starting a family, but nature had decided otherwise. I sympathised with them, because my wife and I had been in the same position; she had fallen pregnant very early on in our marriage, when we were still in the process of getting to know each other. Even so, when the baby arrived, neither my wife nor I would have considered putting the clock back. When I now look at my eldest daughter, more than 30 years after the event, I think of what we would have missed if she had not been born.

It is a Dutch custom to send printed cards to family and friends to announce the happy event of the birth of a baby. This announcement contains the name of the baby and the date of the birth, and it is not unusual to find the quotation of a text or a small poem on such a card. A few weeks ago we received just such an announcement and we were touched to read the following quotation:

Small as you are, so large is the miracle of life.
Until now no one has known you, except God.
He has made us a gift of you.

This card was sent to us by my nephew and his wife who, like the other couple mentioned, had been surprised to learn about the pregnancy so early in their marriage. It had not been planned, though after the initial shock, they had grown used to the idea and happily anticipated the start of their family. Consequently, the quotation on the card was even more touching.

We can only be grateful that the overall plan of Life is not ours to decide. It is not in our hands what happens and when. Life is a great leveller. I explained this to the young couple before she was completely positive that she was pregnant. She had heard about a home-pregnancy test and to cheer them up I told them about some of the old-fashioned pregnancy tests. She phoned me later to tell me that she had used a pregnancy kit and that the result had been positive. She was arranging to make a doctor's appointment. Indeed, the pregnancy was confirmed. We discussed their changing outlook and they began to regard it as a challenge to face up to, and prepare for the changes in their lives brought about by the arrival of a first baby. When that baby arrives life changes for ever. There is an indescribable relationship with the tiny, as yet unknown, embryo to whom you have made a lifelong commitment. Every part of your life will change, from the moment of conception onwards. It is wonderful to see the development of the baby; every day brings some new discovery. There is nothing quite like it.

Admittedly, parenthood is not all sheer pleasure, because it brings with it plenty of problems, and these start all too soon. You are responsible for this small life and you worry if you have done something wrong or forgotten to do something when the baby cries. There are indeed moments when the responsibility weighs almost too heavily. Yet, life would be empty without that little person. Once the baby has arrived, no mother would seriously wish to turn the clock back, even though this is often suggested in jest. Of course, there will be moments of worry, but if you weren't worrying about the baby, or child, you would be worrying about something else. Think of the richness and purpose a child gives to your lives. When I look at my four children, all adults now with a place of their own in life, and in turn looking after children of their own, it is just wonderful to know that this was all part of an overall plan over which we have had little or no control.

The young couple grew used to the idea, and over the months I soon discovered that they still had their dreams, but now these dreams included a third person, a little person. It is wonderful to see a small baby develop into a toddler, to know that you are totally responsible for its care, and to guide it and prepare it for when it starts school, further education and when it goes out into the world. If the right relationship is there, it can be the most rewarding thing in our lives. Never think that because you gave birth to this child and because you brought the child up, that you can keep it for life. My mother used to say that it was wonderful to have children, but always remember that they are only on loan because the day will come when you have to let them flee the nest, and you can only hope that you have prepared them as best you can.

The birth of a baby is an experience which defies description. Most people have fallen in love with their baby even before its birth, and feel very protective towards it. A woman's maternal responses are also normal. That little baby needs you for warmth, food, comfort, security, love and understanding. Special hugs and cuddles are equally beneficial to the baby and the parent. Once a mother has her baby in her arms this maternal feeling will continue to grow and develop. Mothers who have decided to breast-feed their baby, may find that this is not always possible. Listen to the advice of the midwife and if breast-feeding is not successful, then change to the bottle. If you accept this decision, it need not necessarily affect the close relationship you will have with your child. The fact is that you are trying to do the best for your baby, and irrespective of whether you are breast or bottle-feeding, as long as you are happy with the situation, this close relatioinship will not be affected. Don't forget to have little chats with your baby, even though you think it does not respond. The sound of your voice is, in itself, soothing to the baby.

Sometimes the mother is so engrossed in her baby that she forgets to look after herself. If the baby wakes during the night, you may have to find ways of catching up on your sleep at other times. You should take good care of your diet, just as you did when you still carried the baby in your womb. You, too, have the right to be looked after, but always make sure not to close out the father, because he also has the right to develop a relationship of his own with the newborn baby. He must be included in the routine and you may decide to instigate a special time for father and baby, for example, at the nightly bath-time.

The mother must make sure that she undergoes the usual medical examinations after the birth has taken place. Just because you feel well does not mean that you do not need these examinations; they are there for your help and protection. Do not belittle the experience your body has been through, because it is not quite as simple as it is sometimes made out. For some women, the pregnancy and delivery is more demanding than for others. My wife used to have the attitude that if mothers in African countries can give birth in the bush, pick up the baby and walk home, so should she. Well, she almost did, because I remember three days after the birth of our third daughter, I found my wife on her feet working as if nothing had happened. I was rather annoyed with her, because there was no need for it as domestic help had been provided so that she could take it easy.

During the period after the birth you should take extra care of your skin and you would be well advised to consider using some rejuvenating skin-care cream. Often during pregancy, women have a better and more glowing skin, because the body's hormonal balance is different. After the birth, the hormone balance will gradually revert to normal levels and during this period you can do with a little outside help. Sans Soucis has a natural product range that contains a good skin-care programme. Their products are well researched and are highly recommended by their users, which is as good a recommendation as any. Of course, this should be used in combination with a diet rich in fruit and vegetables, and remember to drink plenty of water.

Some women complain about stretch marks and you may be interested to note that Sans Soucis also has a good anti-blemish stick that will help overcome these marks. Let me assure you though, that these marks are more noticeable to you than to anyone else. Also, as a preventative measure during pregnancy, you should rub the body with baby oil every night, and do not forget to include the breasts. Women often think that stretch marks only appear on the hips or stomach, but the thighs can be affected and also the breasts, because they get heavier during the latter stages of pregnancy.

More or less from birth, a baby's nervous system will respond to sound and light. Do some simple reflex exercises with the baby, such as placing your finger in the baby's hand and feel how tightly it grasps it. When you hold the baby upright on your lap, you will be surprised at the strength of its kick, and you must remind yourself that it is not yet strong enough to walk. In truth, the strength is there, but the muscle control is missing. The baby's arms will strike out in reaction to sudden loud noises. Babies love it when you move their little legs up and down and when you place your hand under their feet to gently resist their kicks. Help the baby to discover its arms and hands and see how, at a very young age, it can gaze at its own hands in pure fascination.

Make sure the baby's eyes are clean and if need be wipe them with some cotton-wool and chamomile water, or with boiled water. Your health visitor or nurse at the antenatal clinic will make sure that the umbilical cord is cleanly removed, which should take no longer than ten days or so. Should there be some indication of infection, make sure that the navel is kept clean and dry. Sometimes it is advisable to dab the naval where the umbilical cord is attached with surgical spirit, which will help to dry out the tissue. This makes sense if the umbilical cord takes longer than usual to die off.

Always make sure that the room temperature is neither too hot nor too cold for the baby. Neither extreme is good for the child and do not forget that the baby is not able to tell you when it is uncomfortable; it can only cry, and then you would have to guess why it is crying: hunger, wind, cold, heat, itch, cramp? The ideal room temperature for a baby is between 20–22°C (70–72°F) and, of course, make sure that the baby is not uncovered at night. It is important that the baby's cradle or cot has a firm mattress, because if good care is taken from birth, back problems in later life may be avoided.

It is possible that some babies will develop a little discoloration after a few days, a condition known as physiological jaundice, which is caused by a temporary build-up of bilirubin. If you feed your baby yourself this can quickly be overcome by eating Jerusalem artichokes, or you may prefer to take some Boldocynara – ten drops three times a day after meals.

Once you feel ready, take the baby out for a walk in the pram. You will enjoy it and so will the baby. The pram should have a firm mattress. The baby can be put outside in the garden for its daytime sleep. The pram should, however, be covered by an insect-net to avoid the risk of being stung. Remember that babies do not sleep all day and sometimes actually get bored. They enjoy it if they are placed near a tree so that they can see the leaves and the branches move with the wind. If you take the baby out in the car, make absolutely certain that you have a safe car-seat. When you invest in a baby-seat for the car, check that it has the British Safety Standards seal of approval.

Also, take a little time to decide on the most suitable nappies. Muslin or terry-towelling nappies are rapidly being replaced by disposable nappies. It is important that you decide to use what you and the baby are most happy with. Listen to the advice of other mothers, but always decide for yourself what would suit you and your baby best. Make sure that you do all you can to prevent your baby from developing nappy-rash. Change the baby as soon as possible after wetting or soiling; clean the baby's bottom gently, but thoroughly, with a cleanser especially for that purpose. If possible, leave the baby for a little while without a nappy and, if there is any sign of redness or soreness, St John's Wort Oil will have a soothing effect.

It is always a pleasure to see how most babies enjoy their bath-time. Free from any encumbrances, they will kick out in a playful manner. In the water one's body weight feels different and this is exactly the same for the baby. Most babies love bath-time, but there are a few safety rules to remember. The tub should always be filled with cold water before hot water is added, and never leave the baby alone. If bath-time is interrupted for any reason at all, please make sure that the baby is wrapped up well before you rush to open the door or answer the phone. A lot of congestion in babies is caused by a change in temperature or a draught.

If the baby cries frequently, you may wonder if and when to pick it up. Remember again that the only form of communication a baby has is crying. It becomes very distressed if it is ignored and babies do need a lot of reassurance, so to comfort your baby you must use your intuition. You will get to know your own baby, and you will get to learn his or her different ways of crying. Many babies have a bout of crying at a certain time of the day, evening or night. You will soon recognise the pattern, well before your baby does, because he or she does it instinctively. Remember that this is quite normal and you should not let this upset you.

It is a different matter if the baby does not sleep at all. I need only look at my two youngest granddaughters. One of them (unfortunately for her mother) seems to be very like I was as a toddler, according to my mother. Indeed, my mother has often told me that she never had any peace with me because I would not sleep. My granddaughter is the same and causes her mother considerable problems. She is so over-active and is on the go all the time that I feel very sorry for her mother and father who are up and down with her half the night. Fortunately for her parents, her brother and sister are quite different, because it would be hard to cope with more than one hyperactive child. She is a lively individual and I am sure that it's simply because she just does not want to miss out on anything. My youngest granddaughter is very different: full of life during the day, full of smiles during the day, but when it's bedtime she settles for the night. She is a model of a baby, very balanced, happy and smiling; she eats well and she sleeps well. This merely shows that all babies are different and have very individual character traits, even at this young age. If, at some stage, the baby is unusually distressed and restless, and its usual pattern is disturbed, there is no harm in giving it a small homoeopathic or herbal dosage of Dormeasan – a few drops often do the trick, and this allows the baby to get its much needed sleep.

Seeing new parents with their young baby reminds me of the happy times my wife and I had with the arrival of every one of our children. A baby rapidly learns to listen to the voices of its father and mother, and it is touching to see how quickly a baby learns to focus on the mother's face and how it feels secure and settles comfortably in her arms.

Many young babies have a skin blemish or mark at birth, such as milk spots, strawberry marks, birthmarks or slate-blue patches, and usually these disappear quickly. Strawberry marks – slightly raised, red marks – may initially increase in size, but will usually disappear quite suddenly. For milk spots or other irritations, some Seven Herb Creme will help to rapidly solve the problem.

Cradle cap is common among babies and, contrary to popular belief, it is rarely caused by external factors. It is mostly the result of a heightened sensitivity. In the case of breast-fed babies the cause of cradle cap may well lie in the mother's diet. Unfortunately, mothers are rarely aware of this. Unless this is pointed out, they are generally unaware of the fact that anything eaten, especially medication, finds its way into their milk, and so is passed on to their baby. For example, if the mother is constipated, she may decide to take a laxative and her breast-fed baby suddenly develops diarrhoea. The baby is then treated without success, until bottle-feeding is introduced and the condition is brought under control. This is so unfortunate because the baby is thus deprived of the best food possible, for no other reason than thoughtlessness.

If a baby has cradle cap and is breast-fed, the mother should check her intake of medication and her food. It is not unusual for cradle cap to disappear within days when the mother removes egg whites from her diet. Babies suffering from cradle cap respond well to less fatty food, and the condition will clear up quickly with external applications of Molkosan. This is a whey concentrate that is very effective in the treatment of cradle cap and also for eczema.

After-pains are often experienced during the first few days after the birth, and a salt bath or icepacks can be used. This would not be the first time that I have recommended that women take a packet of frozen peas, wrap it in a towel, and place it on the sore area. Please, always remember that the frozen article should not touch the skin, it must be wrapped in a towel. This usually does the trick. If there is bruising or stitches take some Arnica, either in the form of tincture or tablets. Hamamelis virginiana (witch-hazel) is also very good and should be applied as a poultice. Remember the simple advice for babies who are in pain because of wind. Stand a halved onion for a little while in some hot water and when it has cooled, give the baby half a teaspoon of this extract and I assure you it works like a miracle.

A baby has a lot of growing and developing to do in the first six months of its life and it is fascinating to watch its progress. Watch how it reacts when you clap your hands, or how it reacts to sudden noises. You will take great delight in seeing the first smile and the way it reacts to your voice. You'll be surprised at its strength when it raises its head off your arm or off its pillow. Try not to miss out on anything at this stage of your baby's development because every day brings a new experience. At about the seventh or eighth month it will positively respond to your voice and will be interested in playing with a rattle or a squeaky, soft toy. By this time you will know your baby's favourite routine and sleeping pattern. Notice how it will be desperately trying to raise itself to sit up and take notice of what is going on around it, and it will want to start crawling. It wants to be on the move and it will take note of movements and sounds. I have seen the differences during these months of development with every one of my children. It is so important for fathers and mothers to spend some quality time with the baby during these first few months so that a good relationship can develop. This can be done even if both parents are working.

I remember one young mother who was not especially happy when she realised that she was pregnant and she came to see me after the baby was born. At first I thought that she looked quite angry and when we spoke, she confided in me that she saw the baby as a major intrusion in her life and she was having great problems in accepting it. Also, the pregnancy had left her with stretch marks and she felt that she was less attractive than she had been before the birth. As she had a demanding job, she wanted to go back to work. I prescribed some Jayvee tablets to relieve the tension and some Vitaforce as a tonic. For the stretch marks I told her to use Cellu Ver Cream at night-time, while during the day she should use Sans Soucis Rejuvenating Cream. We discussed her urge to return to work and I pointed out that while she may have a very worthwhile career, she was the most important person in her baby's life and this was a privilege which she should enjoy. I reassured her that when she had re-established the balance in her life she would be more settled. Indeed, within three weeks she was back, on top of the world again, happy with her baby and ready to go to work.

Sometimes the unexpected situations in life, breaking the routine, can have an unsettling effect. I am rather a routine person myself and I fully appreciate that some people struggle to accept changes in their lifestyle. Remember that it is no use getting angry or upset about it; one has no option but to accept the facts, get on with life and enjoy it to the full. If your new arrival is very small you may have to make some adjustments to your expectations. You may be desperate to pick up your baby, but it may not yet be allowed out of the incubator. Even then, there is no reason why you should not consciously begin to develop this precious mother-and-child bond with your baby.

I must stress again the possibility of a hidden allergy in your baby and, in order to prevent the development of unforeseen conditions, you should be aware of this. I have seen it a few times with mothers who were allergic to gluten. There is always a chance that the baby may have inherited this sensitivity and when the baby goes onto solid food the mother should be particularly alert to any changes in the baby's pattern of behaviour.

If the new arrival has colic problems it can be a very tiring time for parents and baby alike. The baby may scream and go red in the face. Attacks may last from two to ten minutes and sometimes come in quick succession. Although this kind of problem is rarely due to the type of food, the possibility of an allergy should be considered. It is often thought that breast-fed babies cannot possibly suffer from this, but if the baby is really sensitive, this may be a reaction to certain foods eaten by the mother, because through her milk, the infant may be affected. Do not get too stressed and try to calm the baby during these bouts of colic. Often fennel water will help to settle things down. Hold the baby and speak soothingly to it to help it through these moments of stress. Worry about the baby's crying will cause considerable stress to the mother. This is understandable, but you must appreciate that this will not last and the baby will grow out of it. When the baby is suffering from colic, you will wonder if it will ever end, but looking back you will realise that it was really only a matter of weeks.

Sensible post-natal care is essential: take extra rest and eat a good and healthy diet to maintain your strength and energy. Do not be ashamed to have a nap during the afternoon, or to go back to bed after your husband has left for work in the morning. Your body will soon let you know when you have done enough, or when you are capable of doing more. If you take good care of yourself, you will also cope better with the baby's demands.

Even during these early days, after the birth of your baby, you may want to start taking some physical exercise. Do not be confused because I have just stressed the importance of taking enough rest.

9

Post-natal Depression

After the excitement that comes with the arrival of a new baby, the mother's initial happiness that all went well is no guarantee against post-natal depression. After all the excitement the mother can still suddenly be hit by this overpowering feeling of depression. Depression can be either the result of psychological worries or because of a nutritional deficiency. If there is the slightest sign of post-natal depression, then it is wise to do something about it immediately.

Post-natal depression affects many women, in a variety of ways: feeling tired or irritable, showing symptoms of a nervous breakdown, even suicidal feelings and a fear of hurting the baby are not unusual. It is estimated that as many as 50 per cent of new mothers suffer from these symptoms to varying degrees, and some doctors suspect that this figure is even higher. Often, a measure of despondency comes over the mother, and she may be tearful, emotional, or unnecessarily pessimistic. Because they are often unable to talk about it, many women feel isolated. Very often, there is a strong sense of not being able to cope with new motherhood. This may also be accompanied by feelings of guilt. Often, a new mother is over-conscientious, and when she persistently complains about her healthy baby, and worries if she is feeding it properly, or is inadequate, the doctor or health visitor needs to pay attention. Irrational fears can be prevalent and although these fears are usually totally unjustified, they may lead to headaches, dizziness, or other physical symptoms which may easily affect the rest of the family. Usually, the husband gets the brunt of it, or the health visitor, which is better because she has come across these symptoms before, and knows not to take it personally. She will be able to advise, whereas the husband may not know what is happening and so may appear to lack understanding. It is good to have someone with whom you can discuss these strange feelings, someone you trust, because some mothers actually become quite aggressive. Fatigue and lack of sleep is one of the most common complaints and I have often had mothers telling me that they felt completely drained of energy. Shakiness, pallor, looking and feeling ill, and being totally despondent, are symptoms of such depression, and a sign that the mother urgently needs help.

What causes such a situation? It may be due to a hormonal imbalance in the body, which takes quite a long time to settle. It could be a social factor, or there may be a previous personality problem. Some women are perfectionists and want to do everything right, but at that particular moment they just cannot cope. They are disappointed by their inability and are loath to admit it. The mother's age, or the number of other children she already has, may be a factor and, indeed, if the mother is slightly older the chances of suffering from depression may be higher. Much depends on where the family lives, particularly if it's in a high-rise flat, or in an isolated rural area. Such feelings of inadequacy and inability to cope with the new responsibility are most prevalent. Long-term use of drugs in the past may also be a factor, as might a Caesarean section or a forceps delivery.

This problem primarily affects those mothers who had a job before the birth of their baby; having been used to colleagues and friends at work, suddenly they are on their own at home with a little baby who is totally dependent on them and requires all their attention. Suddenly, the mother realises that she may have to give up some of her pleasures, and certainly some of her freedom to come and go as she pleased. Her friends are either single or childless, and she may have to decide whether to give up her job, or hand over some of the responsibility to a childminder; and this in turn will aggravate any feelings of guilt she may already have. Sometimes, the realisation suddenly hits her that because she now has a baby she has entered a new phase in her life and is getting older. She will have to be more responsible now there is a baby who depends upon her. Please remember that, although you may have lost some of your freedom, you do not need to have less fun.

Another problem can occur if the father lacks sympathy and understanding. In the first place, he may not have wanted a child, and now feels jealous of all the attention being centred on the baby. Although the mother has given him the most precious gift possible, he feels threatened because the focus of her attention has moved from him onto this helpless little creature. Very often, fathers are also affected by this sudden added responsibility, but they rarely admit to it, because it does not appear to be the manly thing to do. If the father struggles to recognise this trait in himself, he is unlikely to be able to support his wife. I can understand if the woman feels somewhat let down by this, and subsequently takes on the full responsibility herself, even if this is not a very wise move. Mothers who have been faithful in everything will feel this rejection from the husband all the more, and this is often translated into depression.

Sexual relationships sometimes become disrupted after childbirth and, unless the husband is understanding and considerate, the wife can easily become upset. Maybe the baby cries just at the wrong time, or maybe the mother is just too tired by having to tend to the baby. The father's jealousy can make him feel that all he is is merely a provider for mother and child. These feelings should not be allowed to fester, because the longer these go on without proper discussion, the more likely they are to become a pattern for the future.

I have also come across a number of cases where the husband was no longer interested in having sex with his wife after she had given birth, and this, quite understandably, caused major marital problems. Suddenly, the man regards his wife in a different light and he finds it difficult to recognise her in her new role as the playmate he once desired. This demonstrates how the mental changes, which take place in a woman's mind when her life has changed so much, also affect the man. I should point out that it is also true that some women are taken aback by the way their husband has taken to their baby, even though beforehand he did not seem to want to be closely involved.

There are other social factors that can play a part in post-natal depression, and it is wise to be alert to these and even to read up about them beforehand, so that some of the early warning signs may be recognised, and help obtained before things get out of hand. Women should know that they can get help. There is no need to feel you have to be infallible. Please take your health visitor or your doctor into your confidence, or mention it at the post-natal clinic. Never be afraid to ask questions, and try to involve the father as much as possible. Sometimes, you may be able to discuss some of your feelings with a friend or your mother, or someone you feel comfortable with. You will soon discover that you are not alone in experiencing these feelings, and you are no less a mother or wife because of them. By facing the facts you may well prevent some of your guilt feelings from getting out of hand.

Whatever you do, always try to share your feelings with someone whose opinion you respect. Please do not keep it bottled up or feel obliged to sort it out yourself. If you have these feelings of inadequacy, make sure that you get plenty of sleep and put some time aside to make yourself look pretty; this will give you much needed confidence. Do not feel guilty if you get the urge to read a good book while the washing-up is still in the sink waiting to be done. You are entitled to some time for yourself and just because you have become a mother, does not mean that you have lost any right to this entitlement. There is no doubt that because you have become a mother your life has changed, but make sure that it is you who decides which changes are acceptable to you. Do not let others impose these upon you. It is up to you and, hopefully, together with your husband, you will find a new routine that includes this helpless little person who has come into your family. Recognition and appreciation of these changes are of prime importance because awareness will help make you cope.

Taking the baby for a walk will give you some of the necessary physical exercise in the fresh air which will do both you and the baby much good. Do not feel guilty if you want to leave the baby with your husband, mother or a friend just so that you can go for a swim, or an exercise class, or meet some friends. Although the responsibility of the newborn baby is yours, this need not be interpreted as your life being put on hold. Your carefree years may be over in a sense, but just because you have become a mother does not automatically mean that you are no longer a person in your own right. Never lose sight of this.

Some mothers tell me that although they wanted the baby desperately, and they have willingly given up their job for the baby, they now feel very lonely. Of course, this can be a problem, but you will find that because of your different circumstances, you now move in other circles. You may become friendly with other mothers you meet at the antenatal clinic, and you will feel comfortable with them because they are most likely experiencing the same feelings you do. Therefore, you may find it easier to share your experiences with them, because they can relate to your problems. The health visitor will also point out that your experiences are not new. Apart from everything else, it will keep you busy developing a comfortable routine for yourself and your baby.

Such problems are more common after a difficult delivery, or if there were already feelings of lethargy or a persistent tiredness before the delivery. Suddenly, when the post-natal depression hits the mother, she feels isolated and lonely. Make sure that these feelings are not aggravated by a nutritional deficiency. Watch your diet carefully and make sure that you eat the right things, because that is where your strength will come from. This is as important after the birth as it was during pregnancy.

If you fear that you are on the road to some form of post-natal depression, first of all take a vitamin B-Complex supplement, and usually I also advise taking a Zinc supplement. I have found that post-natal depression is often quickly overcome when a chemical deficiency is rectified. Herbal teas, as mentioned in the chapter entitled Herbal Remedies, may also be of help. Remember that alternative medicine offers many remedies which are infinitely preferable to any long-term orthodox treatment of anti-depressants and hormones, or psychotherapy. I am sure the key to recovery lies mostly within oneself. Therefore, prior education and awareness of potential problems is a much better preparation for the demands of parenthood and will help you to retain your joy and enthusiasm.

I have specifically mentioned the long-term use of anti-depressants and hormones, because I was shocked when I read the results of a recent survey by the Institute of Child Health in Bristol. Apparently 50 per cent of pregnant women admitted taking Paracetamol even though the effect of this drug on a developing baby is unknown. The survey monitored 1,100 pregnant women in the Avon area and examined the health of their babies as they grew up, in order to find out what factors influenced the children's health. First analyses have shown that, during the first 18 weeks of pregnancy, 54 per cent of the women had taken Paracetamol tablets, compared with only 4 per cent taking Aspirin tablets. The head of the project, Dr Jean Golding, thought this percentage was incredibly high and contacted the manufacturers to try and find out why so many women took Paracetamol. However, she did stress that there is no scientific evidence that Paracetamol poses a risk to unborn babies, and pointed out that just possibly it could do more harm if mothers-to-be suffered pain. The article continued:

Drugs and Pregnancy
Doctors in France gave either half an aspirin tablet or one dummy tablet a day to 300 women at risk of having abnormally small babies when they were 18 weeks pregnant. The babies in the aspirin group were on average 8oz (225g) heavier than those in the dummy group, and neither mother nor baby experienced any extra side-effects. A huge international study of aspirin in pregnancy is now underway, but early data on 3,000 women suggests that there were no ill effects.

However, I feel that there is still some doubt about this and, therefore, anything that might possibly be harmful is better avoided. When I read in the article that 50 per cent of pregnant women were taking Paracetamol I shivered. Although there may not be any side-effects, I find it hard to accept that such extensive use of painkillers should take place during pregnancy. One can never be too careful with the use of any medication in these circumstances and there has been a great deal of adverse publicity on the subject.

It is much better and safer to take a natural remedy, and a number of possible options have been mentioned in the earlier chapters on homoeopathic and herbal medicine. When you recognise symptoms such as apathy, reduced energy and concentration, excessive tiredness, headaches, self-pity, phobias, lack of appetite, sleeplessness or even suicidal thoughts, first check that the diet is adequate and not lacking in any essential ingredients. A wholesome diet should contain foods that are rich in minerals, vitamins and trace elements. The latter constituents will often have to be supplemented in another form. Often, a daily supplement of one or two tablets of Health Insurance Plus will pay off handsomely. This supplement can be safely taken over long periods and offers all the main antioxidant nutrients, calcium, magnesium, and a wide range of supplementary vitamins and minerals. Please note, however, that this supplement is recommended for use *after* the birth and should not be taken *during* pregnancy.

In the herbal field, I can wholeheartedly recommend some supplementary alfalfa, pineapple, ginseng, passiflora, or St John's Wort. Extra vitamin B12 is very important in cases of post-natal depression. As a soothing herbal preparation I have often recommended the use of the JayVee tablets. These tablets contain a blend of natural source substances known to have soothing properties including the herb valerian, crataegus (hawthorn), humulus lupulus (hops), passiflora, melissa (lemon balm) and zinc; all of which combine well with valerian. In most cases, this has been very helpful, but again it should be remembered that this is recommended for use *after* childbirth and not *during* pregnancy. If necessary, this prescription can be backed up by an additional tonic and for this I usually recommend Dr Vogel's Vitaforce.

TriMax is a potent remedy devised specifically to counteract indefinite complaints during post-natal depression. Some women find it hard to confide and share their emotions. Feelings of guilt, being unloved, and worthlessness, are often the classic signs. Because they are so reluctant to come to terms with their condition, a potent remedy such as TriMax (maximum dose: two tablets three times daily) will help to overcome this psychological barrier, and the patient will be more inclined to disclose the problems, and as such be impelled to confront their worries. Often they are reluctant to recognise the problem, because they feel such a failure. Depression can be a prison created by the sufferer, yet if only they can find the strength to turn the key, to discuss their problems, they will be able to come to terms with the situation and be happy again. Life is too short to be locked in a cage of depression for long.

I remember meeting an attractive young mother who was the daughter of a very successful doctor. She had asked her father, as well as others, for help, and finally turned to alternative medicine. We had a long chat and I pointed out that blood circulatory problems were often at the root of this condition. Therefore, I prescribed Hyperisan, a remedy that has often been helpful in unlocking depression. I also prescribed Avena sativa, which is an oat extract, and within two weeks she was beginning to feel better. Because she did not sleep very well I suggested a course of JayVee tablets and, to counter her lack of enthusiasm and bring back her normal *joie de vivre*, I prescribed Ginsavita and Imuno-Strength. These remedies definitely helped her turn the corner and I was so pleased to see a change in her. Her husband came with her at her next appointment and they told me how happy they were with their baby, and that they were so grateful for her return to her usual self.

Another case I remember was a mother who suffered from post-natal depression caused by grief. She was upset about a friend who died during her pregnancy and I was sorry that she had not come to me then. However, I prescribed Ignatia 30X and this changed her condition overnight. It is marvellous that a constitutional homoeopathic remedy can affect such a major turnaround. It is sad that the enthusiastic, loving and happy emotions experienced at the birth of a baby do not always last. The confusion in the baby's first few months is quite understandable, but with determination and trust involving both partners, this can be such a happy time. Please don't allow anything to distract you and jeopardise your happiness. Just think of that wonderful creation lying there in its crib, the result of both your efforts, your love and your understanding, and the happiness that it will bring you in the future.

10

Teething Problems

The rate of development in babies or infants varies enormously. Some are quick to walk, speak, or teethe. My daughters were all quick to walk, but all had considerable problems when teething. Teething can be a fraught experience for both parents and infants alike. Some sail through this experience, while others are irritable and irksome for weeks on end, and exhausting to the parents, whose sleep is too often disturbed. No sooner has one tooth come through when there seems to be a repeat performance and parents and babies have to go through it all again. The baby is fortunate in that it can make up for its lost sleep at any time it likes, unlike the parents. Teething, although painful in itself, usually affects the baby's motions and can bring about a sore bottom. This can be a stressful time and the child can be very grumpy.

It is remarkable how fast a child grows into an interesting little person. The change from breast- or bottle-feeding to drinking from a cup is seen as a major milestone, but this is nothing like feeling or seeing the first tooth appear. The gums can be sore for quite some time before the tooth actually appears and when you see the inflamed gums, you cannot help but feel sorry for the little mites. A teething ring is often helpful, because it eases some of the irritation of the gums. It seems that one baby in every 2,000 already has a little tooth at birth, sometimes this may be loose, but not always. This is not as strange as it may sound, because six months prior to the actual birth the teeth are already present in the mouth of the foetus.

With this in mind the general advice to top up calcium intake during pregnancy makes perfect sense. Not only is it important for the mother, but equally so for the foetus. This foetus will take its required calcium from the mother, and unless the mother makes sure that her diet contains added calcium, or takes a supplement to achieve this, she will suffer a calcium deficiency and she will notice a drastic deterioration in her own teeth after the birth.

The baby will get his first teeth at approximately seven months, and may be three and a half before all 20 milk-teeth are present. This again varies according to the individual rate of development. This teething process in babies can be accompanied by a varied pattern of symptoms, which may range from skin problems, a rise in temperature, diarrhoea, or bronchitis, to minor fits or convulsions. Old manuscripts on folk and herbal medicine are full of advice about teething problems, and it is consoling to know that mothers have always struggled with their child's complaint.

In the sixteenth century a doctor hit on the idea of cutting a baby's gums in an effort to minimise its discomfort when teething. Prior to that, a tooth powder was used during the most stressful times but, fortunately, this habit was discontinued because the powder contained mercury, which would not have done the baby any good at all. In fact, it would slowly poison the child.

The cutting-teeth or incisors usually appear first in the lower jaw, and then in the upper jaw. The cutting of the eye-teeth or canine teeth happens long before the incisors appear. Again, this varies from infant to infant. Last to arrive are the back teeth or the molars, and the child's teeth may not be complete until it is in its fourth year.

These teeth are replaced by a more permanent set of teeth in later life, but even so it should be understood that the milk-teeth can be adversely affected by too many sweets and sugars in the diet. Remember that teeth are an investment for the future, and if the milk-teeth are decayed it is likely that the permanent set of teeth will have been affected. A friend of one of my daughters used to give her baby a dummy dipped in honey when she settled him down for the night and when he woke up during the night, to help him settle again. When she was warned that this was unwise, she claimed that honey was a natural product and therefore could not possibly be harmful. However, the honey that covered this little dummy was allowed to mix with the infant's saliva and remained there for the rest of the night. Some time later, the mother was shocked to see that the child's milk-teeth were severely decayed and the enamel coating partially absent. It must have been an awful sight to see a young toddler with blackened teeth, and she most definitely learned her lesson. There is no doubt that, although her intentions were good, the outcome was absolutely disastrous.

Be warned; use your common sense and follow the professional's advice. Many conditions would be discovered sooner if the mother had had the baby checked by an osteopath, as I suggested in the chapter on cranial osteopathy. The structure of the facial part of the skull is very complex. The greater part of the hard palate, or roof of the mouth, is formed by the maxilla and the palatine bones quite often appear as relatively small bridges with numerous connections to the cranial bones, and these should all work in harmony. If the maxilla is knocked into an internal rotation, a painful condition can occur and, although this condition is not very common, it is possible that it may be hereditary. It can also be evidence of a forceps delivery, or a prolonged birth. At a later stage, this can manifest itself in breathing difficulties, sinus problems, catarrh, lack of visual acuteness, and crowded and/or irregular teeth. Children's teeth can easily be overcrowded and this internal check-up may well prevent secondary dentitional placement problems. The terminal teeth will have great difficulty in coming through, as the first teeth have not left enough space. If the child breathes through the mouth, or sucks its thumb a lot, it may well need braces on the teeth, or the baby-teeth may have to be removed by a dentist. These abnormal situations could have been rectified at an early stage by an osteopath, and the trauma of tooth extraction at a young age could therefore have been avoided.

It should be noted that there are a number of extremely effective homoeopathic remedies for the pain and discomfort of teething. In the first instance, I would recommend the use of Chamomilla, which will help reduce the irritability, the flushing of the cheeks, and which also has a soothing effect. If the gums are really sore and the infant also suffers from diarrhoea, Mercurius 6C is helpful and Aconite 30C should be recommended for acute pain and high temperature, Nux 6C is beneficial if the teething process causes constipation and straining when passing a motion. If Propolis Gelee is gently rubbed onto the gums before the infant is put down for the night, the baby is more likely to have an undisturbed night. Sometimes it makes sense to use a combined homoeopathic remedy; Nelson's Teeth Formula has proved very useful during such difficult times. Again, if the baby is restless and frequently wakes during the night because of teething problems, it can do no harm to give it three to five drops of Dormeasan before it goes to sleep, which will help it sleep, and will also bring welcome relief to the parents.

11

Conception and Contraception

A few years ago a young Dutch couple arrived at my clinic in Scotland. They had heard of me and knew that I had made a special study on the subject of multiple sclerosis. They were an interesting couple and we spent a very pleasant evening together. I was, however, slightly mystified when they told me that she had been positively diagnosed as suffering from multiple sclerosis. Somehow I had my doubts, even though she was barely able to walk and spent most of her time in a wheelchair. The next day I performed several tests, which all proved to be inconclusive. Finally, after asking repeatedly if she took any medication, she admitted to taking the contraceptive pill. I am not sure if she had involuntarily tried to hide this fact from me, or positively she just did not regard the contraceptive pill as a form of medication. In any case, after I learned about this I performed a few allergy tests, because I have noticed that very occasionally the side-effects from the contraceptive pill can be similar to some of the symptoms of multiple sclerosis. It was then that I discovered that she was allergic to the contraceptive pill.

I prescribed a homoeopathic nosode to the contraceptive pill and she suffered a very severe reaction. Her husband phoned me in the middle of the night to let me know that she had a very high temperature and I congratulated him because this proved that the nosode was taking effect. He was very worried and asked me to come to the hotel that night, but I told him that it could safely wait until the next morning. My suspicions were correct and her high temperature was a reaction to the homoeopathic nosode. When she returned to the Netherlands, she was able to walk again unaided. Her neurologist in the Netherlands was extremely interested and phoned to ask about the treatment I had prescribed. I explained that in some rare cases an allergy to the contraceptive pill may cause symptoms similar to those associated with multiple sclerosis, but that this did not in fact prove that the woman was actually suffering from multiple sclerosis. She only displayed the symptoms of this disease.

The crucial point to this little story is that it raises the question of whether the contraceptive pill is as safe as one is made to believe. An allergy to the contraceptive pill, and the same principle indeed applies to HRT (Hormone Replacement Therapy), is rather exceptional but, nevertheless, in all my years in practice this was not the first time I had come across this condition. For some of my patients these problems have been rather drastic and even life-threatening.

In this chapter it is not my intention to judge the use of contraceptive methods, as this is primarily the responsibility of the two partners involved. What I must say, however, is that if one thinks about becoming pregnant, stop all oral means of contraception and the use of any IUD (Intra-Uterine Device) *three months* prior to the start of any planned pregnancy.

There are some contraceptives which, I fear, are detrimental to a woman's health. It is a very personal and difficult subject, but both partners need to be informed of the advantages and the disadvantages of their chosen contraceptive method. Without the total picture they will not be able to make a balanced decision. On the whole, my advice would be that the more natural the means of contraception used, the less risk this will pose to the woman's health. If a decision has been reached and the choice is in favour of the contraceptive pill, please consider reducing the risk by taking some dietary supplements. Also, you should be aware that the risk factor increases for females who smoke, when the incidence of heart and artery problems becomes significantly higher.

I have often heard the argument sway towards the contraceptive pill because, as a means of contraception, it is more reliable than any other, even though others are potentially less damaging to a woman's health; the withdrawal method, for example. A great deal of the control rests with the male partner here, and even then, this method is still not totally reliable because sperm can escape prior to ejaculation. As IUDs go; the 'coil', a small flexible device made largely of plastic, needs to be professionally fitted, and over the years I have seen a number of patients who have fallen pregnant when they thought they were safe because they used the coil. This method is more suitable for women who have already had children.

Then there are are injectable contraceptives, which contain a large amount of progesterone, injected into the muscle for slow release into the body. These jabs are designed to prevent the release of eggs from the ovaries.

Then, of course, there is the most drastic decision of all; sterilisation. I would find it impossible to estimate the number of people who have consulted me because they regretted this step. Sterilisation should be regarded as irreversible and, therefore, a great deal of thought should be given to this method of contraception, as either partner may live to seriously regret their decision. This applies to sterilisation of the female as well as the male. In certain circumstances the latter may be reversed, but this cannot be guaranteed and often leads to problems and complications.

Social factors should certainly be considered, but not at the expense of major health hazards. It is impossible to over-emphasise how important it is to consider carefully which contraceptive method is most suitable for you and your partner, and you should always bear in mind that your circumstances may well change.

I have already mentioned that the risks associated with the contraceptive pill are increased if the woman smokes. It should also be pointed out that it is generally not advisable to use the pill beyond the age of 35. In cases of high blood pressure, diabetes, migraines, circulation, gallbladder, liver or heart problems the contraceptive pill should not be used.

Unfortunately, there are no homoeopathic or herbal contraceptives, but there are many techniques which can be used as a means of contraception, and the methods which follow can be used both as a way of avoiding, or of achieving, a pregnancy.

Women who have a normal menstruation cycle are fertile for a short period only, which is around the ovulation time – the days in the middle of the cycle. There are three reliable methods to discover when you are ovulating; the temperature method, the calendar method and the Billings method. As soon as menstruation starts, a new egg cell ripens in the ovary. It takes about 13 days before this ripened egg cell starts its journey to the womb, where it can be fertilised. If fertilisation does not take place, menstruation will start after approximately 14 or 15 days. That period of 15 days is fairly consistent. The length of menstruation, and of the ripening of the egg, indicates the timing of the ovulation. In some women this can change from one month to another, while other women have a very regular cycle. Fertilisation is not only possible on the day the ripened egg starts its journey, because the male sperm can stay alive in the uterus for at least 48 hours. Therefore, sexual intercourse two days prior to the egg reaching the womb can still lead to pregnancy. Moreover, the eggs can be fertilised up to 12 hours after ovulation and it is always possible that the egg's journey starts earlier or later than expected. Fertilisation is therefore possible four days before the expected ovulation and three days afterwards; including the actual day of ovulation. That means that there is a total of eight unsafe days during the middle of the month.

All these factors should be taken into account if you decide to use the calendar method as an aid to conception or a means of contraception. A menstruation calendar needs careful administration and calculation, taking into account the starting dates of the last two menstruations. It would be better still if you kept a record going further back, because that way you will know if your periods are regular. Once you have worked out the duration of the shortest and longest cycle you will be able to calculate when your unsafe period is. Remember, when making your calculations, that you must start counting from the very first day of your present period.

The temperature method is based on the fact that the body temperature in the second half of the menstrual cycle is 0.3–0.5°C higher than during the first half of the cycle. This increase occurs one or two days after ovulation. This information can then be used to calculate your safe and unsafe dates. Bear in mind that there may, of course, be another reason for a slight increase in temperature, such as a sleepless night or an infection.

You should be meticulous in noting down these temperatures, which should be measured at the same time every morning before getting up. Use the same thermometer, because here again there might be a very slight variation. It is easiest to record these temperatures, day in, day out, on a sheet of squared or graph paper so that a graph can be compiled for easier reading. If you decide to take this information to your doctor for discussion, remember that you should have records for at least three consecutive months.

I have had very good feedback from a number of my patients on the Billings Ovulation method. If this is followed correctly the risk of pregnancy is greatly reduced and, like the calendar method and the temperature method, this contraceptive method does not require any unnatural ingredients which could have side-effects.

The Billings Ovulation method is based on a special version of periodic abstinence. As you may not be familiar with this method I will give you the details later in the following chapter. The great benefit of this method is that it is a natural form of family planning which can help you to either become pregnant, or to avoid pregnancy. It is also harmless and reliable. There is no cost involved, no drugs or appliances to buy, and, moreover, periodic abstinence has no detrimental effect on one's health. You may also find it worthwhile to consult a book called, *The Billings Method – Controlling Fertility Without Drugs or Devices*, written by Evelyn Billings and Ann Westmore.

The Billings Ovulation Method of natural family planning is a method of avoiding or of achieving pregnancy, based on observing and recording the natural mucus secretion which every woman of child-bearing age notices coming from the vagina for a few days some two weeks before menstruation, from puberty right through to the menopause. It can be used at all times during a woman's fertile life, including after childbirth, during breast-feeding, and in the pre-menopausal years. Whether the cycles are regular or irregular, it has been found to be a reliable method.

Scientific studies indicated that with proper instruction and motivation, this method is 98 per cent effective, and also much safer than the most popular artificial or chemical methods. When I queried the very few failures of contraception that I have learned about, it somehow transpired that the instructions had not been properly adhered to, and also that the women concerned had not bothered to read the book. All the advice on this method is very professionally presented and explained.

The Mucus Patterns of Fertility and Infertility

Explanation:
1. Every woman of child-bearing age notices that at some time between her menstruations she has a white or colourless vaginal discharge of what is called mucus.
2. This mucus discharge is not an abnormality. It is an indication of good health and tells the woman that now is the time when an act of intercourse may cause pregnancy.
3. When the mucus begins to appear, the vulva feels sticky and the mucus looks opaque. Next, it becomes slippery and may look clear and stretchy, like the raw white of an egg. Then it becomes dry or sticky and usually stops altogether. Some women notice the slippery feeling without actually seeing any mucus.
4. The most fertile days are those when the vulva feels slippery and for two or three days afterwards.
5. Sometimes a little bleeding occurs between one menstruation and the next.

Rules if you want to have a child:

1. Pay attention to a slippery feeling on the vulva, and watch for the days of stretchy, slippery mucus. These may not occur in every cycle.
2. The best chance of having a child is likely to occur if intercourse takes place on the days when the woman is most aware of the slippery feeling produced by the mucus.
3. The husband's fertility may be enhanced at the same time by a rest from intercourse for a few days beforehand.

Rules if you do not wish to have a child:

1. Avoid intercourse during menstruation.
2. Avoid intercourse on days when the mucus is present and for at least three days afterwards.
3. Avoid intercourse on days of slight bleeding, and for at least three days afterwards, when bleeding occurs between one menstruation and the next.

Instructions (on the Billings Method and on compiling a chart, with boxes numbered 1–35 from left to right):

1. All genital contact should be avoided for the first month if correct information is to be obtained.
2. Start to record today in the chart. Leave a gap in which to record the date of the last menstruation, birth, miscarriage or last pill. Write the date of the start of the record. Each evening, record the observations made during the day, using a mark of the appropriate colour or symbol as described in paragraphs 4–7.
3. When the next menstruation begins, write in the date and the day of the week in the margin on the left. Continue writing the names of the following weekdays in compartments drawn across the page.
4. To record the first day of menstruation, draw a red mark in the first compartment covering the name of the weekday. On each successive day of menstruation draw another red mark in the next compartment. Note the possible occurrence of mucus during the final days of menstruation, when the bleeding is slight. If any mucus occurs write a description of it in the compartment beneath, note the feeling that it produces as it leaves the body and its visual characteristics, if there is enough to be seen.
5. When menstruation stops, and there is a sensation of dryness in the genital area around the vagina (vulva), and no mucus is visible, make a green mark in the next compartment.

6. Continue with the green marks each day until the feeling of dryness stops. These dry days are infertile days, unless preceded by mucus.
7. When the sensation of dryness has gone, this means that the mucus has begun. Now you may like to make a white mark or draw a little baby in the relative compartment.
8. A dry day may be difficult to recognise if intercourse has occurred on the previous evening. Avoid genital contact and record the day with a white mark or a corresponding signal.
9. Over the next few days the vulva usually feels sticky or damp, and the mucus looks cloudy.
10. As ovulation approaches, the type of mucus changes; it usually becomes clearer and stretches without breaking, like the raw white of an egg; the amount may increase or decrease, and sometimes it is tinged with some blood. The mucus now has fertile signs. Close to ovulation there may be pain in the side. Even before ovulation the stretchiness of the mucus may disappear, the amount diminish and the mucus may become cloudy, but a sensation of lubrication persists in the genital area around the vagina because the mucus continues to be slippery and smooth, indicating the time of maximum fertility. Do not examine the vagina internally.
11. The last day of the slippery, lubricative mucus is the peak symptom.
12. On the first day past the peak symptom, the mucus will become opaque or sticky or stop altogether so that you may feel dry. Now you can indicate with an 'X' the day on which you think you experienced the peak symptom. If another day of slippery, lubricative mucus occurs after this, you have misjudged the peak and will need to mark the record again. If the slippery feeling continues, you have not passed the peak, even if the mucus has become cloudy, or can no longer be seen.
13. Continue to draw a baby each day until three days past the peak symptom. If the mucus has become sticky and opaque, draw a yellow baby. If the mucus has gone and the vulva is dry, draw a green baby.
14. If, at any time, mucus reappears, record it and describe it.
15. On the fourth day past the peak symptom, you are again infertile. From now on every day of the cycle is infertile, even if some opaque, non-stretchy, mucus is present. Continue to record at the end of each day, using a green mark if no mucus is felt or seen, and a yellow pen if mucus is present.

16. The next menstruation should occur some 11–16 days after the peak symptom. When it arrives, verify the accuracy of your identification of the peak by checking this interval.

17. When this next menstruation begins, start a new line on the record the same way as before. Remember to mark the record in red at the end of each day.

18. Each cycle has its own pattern. Do not expect it to match any other cycle.

19. It is wise to record on the chart the last act of intercourse ahead of the 'baby days', and the first act after they are ended. Any error of application will then be quickly observed, and not be repeated.

20. The Basic Infertile Pattern: before ovulation in some long cycles, during breast-feeding, near the menopause, etc. There may be mucus every day or a succession of three or four or even more days when mucus is present, separated by days when there is no mucus. When there is mucus every day, that mucus which remains the same, day after day after day, is a Basic Infertile Pattern, just as in other cycles the dry days before ovulation constitute the Basic Infertile Pattern. When dry days and mucus days both occur intermittently, and the mucus is the same whenever it is present during two weeks of observation, you now have a combined Basic Infertile Pattern of dry days and mucus days. Record the Basic Infertile Pattern of mucus with a yellow marker. Record any change from the Basic Infertile Pattern in white, and count three days after return to the Basic Infertile Pattern. In cycles of average length three cycles should be studied in order to confirm that the Basic Infertile Pattern of dry days or mucus is the same day after day, cycle after cycle.

21. In using the Billings Ovulation Method to avoid pregnancy, intercourse ahead of ovulation must be confined to days on which the Basic Infertile Pattern has been recognised, so intercourse should be delayed until the evening. Abstinence is necessary on days of heavy bleeding during the menstrual period, and also on days when there has been a change from the Basic Infertile Pattern and for three days after it returns. When ovulation occurs, infertility returns on the fourth day past the peak and it is no longer necessary for intercourse to be confined to the evening, nor avoided on the next day.

Abortion

Throughout the ages abortion has been an emotive subject and the amount of money which has changed hands with back-street abortionists, or been paid over in private clinics, has been astronomical. Usually, this was done to maintain secrecy because of the social stigma attached to being single and pregnant, and often the parents of the girl in such an unenviable position either deserted her or forced her to have the unwanted pregnancy terminated.

It is a good thing that nowadays there is an increased awareness of this post-abortion syndrome and that there are groups where women, who have been psychologically hurt by a terminated pregnancy, irrespective of whether this was planned or spontaneous, can get help. The counsellors are familiar with the syndrome and often are people who have had to make this difficult decision themselves at some time or another, and so they are in an excellent position to help others.

There is a book, *Women Hurt by Abortion*, which anyone who has been in a position where they have had to decide for or against an abortion, or anyone at present in that position, should read. Also, *The Secret Life of the Unborn Child* is a remarkable and controversial book that looks at life before birth, and should be read by anyone who has been pressurised or is being pressurised into a pro-abortion decision.

Post-abortion syndrome can express itself in a number of ways: emotional numbness, sleeplessness, back pain, sexual difficulties, eating disorders, preoccupation, lack of concentration, psychosomatic symptoms, violence, repression of emotions, self-punishment, and so on. For men, the decision in favour of an abortion can also have great psychological impact.

Sadly, I have had my fair share of patients who have suffered from post-abortion syndrome. Some of them made their decision for the very best of reasons, and certainly not all of them regretted it, yet they all had a peculiar sadness about them when they referred to it.

12

Complications

From the very moment my wife told me that she was pregnant I worried. My wife, fortunately, is a realist and keeps both feet firmly on the ground, but sometimes my imagination gets the better of me. Therefore, during all her pregnancies I worried and imagined all the things which could go wrong. In the medical profession we see our share of sad cases and I had to remind myself that these constituted only a small percentage, and that the large majority of babies are healthy at birth. Nevertheless, I was always very happy when the new baby arrived once I had checked that all the limbs were there and that there were no obvious signs of deformity.

When I was still studying, my sister-in-law, who had two healthy children, gave birth to a baby with a major skull deformity. I was absolutely devastated, because in my naïvety I had never expected to actually come across such a situation. The baby girl lived for only four days, and even that appeared to be a miracle to me. Looking at the poor little mite was so upsetting because one side of her head lacked any covering of bone tissue. Every time my wife was pregnant this picture would flash back into my mind, and I have always been extremely grateful that God has given us four healthy children, and at the last count, five healthy grandchildren.

So, I worried unnecessarily, but in that I am not alone. Some people worry so much that it ruins the experience of being pregnant and carrying a new life, which should be such a happy time, a time for preparation, and a time for sharing the anticipation of a new life together with your partner. I remember one such patient whose worries far outweighed her pleasure at being pregnant, and I was able to sympathise with her. Because of this understanding I was able to help her come to terms with her fears, and, as is most often the case, her fears eventually proved to be unfounded because she gave birth to a healthy baby boy.

Nevertheless, complications can never be ruled out. It is established that in the UK approximately 60,000 women per year fail to carry their baby full-term and therefore miscarry. It is always a sad experience, and I remember my mother's sadness when she told me that she had lost a baby through miscarriage prior to my birth. I learned that such an experience leaves a deep psychological scar, because the loss of an unborn child is very similar to the loss of an actual child.

We have come to expect that little can go wrong during pregnancy because medical science has become so advanced, and yet, why a woman should miscarry and spontaneously abort a foetus remains something of a mystery. About 20 per cent of all pregnancies end in miscarriage and it is often thought that this is nature's way of dealing with an imperfect foetus. I quote from a magazine article on this subject: 'It's like being struck by lightning and it's against all odds that it will happen a second time.' If the mother has a medical condition, of course it may happen again, but science has come a very long way. I had a female patient who had had three miscarriages, and yet she went on to carry the fourth baby full-term, and two more after that.

Although a miscarriage is initially regarded as a mystery, often, at a later stage, it can be linked to some incident or shock, emotional upset or trauma. Too often such instances can cause the loss of a foetus before the twenty-eighth week of the pregnancy. There are some homoeopathic remedies that may help in such circumstances. If there is early bleeding or pain, you must inform your doctor or midwife immediately. It may be reassuring to know that it is safe to take Arnica 30C, and in the event of a steady loss of blood, take Ipecacuanha 30C. For abdominal cramps, take Pulsatilla, and when very tense two tablets of Neuroforce may be taken twice daily. In the case of a threatened miscarriage or occasional bleeding during pregnancy, take Hamamelis virg (witch-hazel) – ten drops three times a day – together with three tablets of Urticalcin.

If the foetus dies in the womb it is inevitable that there will be a discharge, usually scanty, brown blood. Women with a history of previous miscarriages need to be especially careful during the first three months of pregnancy. I have already mentioned that Arnica may safely be taken during the first few months and it is also very important to take a complex vitamin preparation, such as Health Insurance Plus, and, in the case of anaemia, it is advisable to take a remedy such as Viralplex.

Probably the most common complaint is morning-sickness. It has always amazed me how my wife was affected by this and I remember that during her first pregnancy she could not bear the smell of a certain brand of soap, even if it was still in its wrapping. At the slightest whiff of this particular brand of soap she would immediately react and go off-colour. During other pregnancies different tastes or smells would upset her. I remember that my mother told me that she had a fierce reaction to cotton-wool. Most women will notice an unusual aversion or reaction to a specific object during their pregnancy.

First-time mothers usually experience nausea or sickness during the first months of pregnancy. There are a number of ways to cure this, such as eating small and more frequent meals, avoiding greasy foods, and quite a few of my patients have been greatly helped by using some of the acupressure points as outlined in my book *Body Energy*, and also some homoeopathic remedies, such as Nux vomica or Pulsatilla and the one I most frequently prescribe, Nat. Mur 6C. Some early pregnancies are accompanied not only by sickness, but also by dizziness. The best cure for this is the homoeopathic tablet, Vertigo Heel. In severe cases, drink some hot water with a little lemon juice at regular intervals.

A number of things can go wrong at any stage of the pregnancy. Miscarriages after the first three months often indicate that there is something wrong with the mother and a medical check-up in early pregnancy is essential. If you do have a miscarriage, follow your doctor's advice and have a thorough medical check, which may help to establish why the miscarriage took place, and avoid the same thing happening again in the future. Around 50 per cent of all early miscarriages stem from chromosomal abnormalities in the foetus. The most common type occurs when the foetus has an extra chromosome, which usually results in Down's syndrome.

Named after John Langdon Down, who first described it in 1866, the condition results from a chromosomal abnormality. But the cause of this condition was not discovered until 1959, when medical researchers found that the cells of those affected had too many chromosomes – 47 instead of 46. Even now, scientists do not know why this extra chromosome develops. One possibility is that a deviation occurs during the first stage of sperm or egg formation, but it is also possible that a deviation develops after fertilisation. Most doctors have their own thoughts on the matter, but no one is absolutely certain.

People with Down's syndrome share certain physical characteristics. Their eyes slope up at the outer corners, they have folds of skin on either side of the nose, are of short stature, have small facial features, a large tongue, a flattening at the back of the head and broad, short hands. These physical signs are evident at birth, and usually become more pronounced as the child grows. As well as the physical characteristics, they are prone to heart defects or intestinal problems, such as duodenal atresia (a narrowing or blocking in the duodenum), often already present at birth. They are also prone to chest infections. In the past, this often meant they had short life-spans. It was rare for Down's syndrome children to survive much beyond their teenage years. Today, early surgery can rectify some of the problems, and the development of antibiotic treatment can eliminate infections. Although exact statistics are not available, it is estimated that the average life-expectancy is now around 50.

It appears that, on average, three babies are born every day in Britain with Down's syndrome. The likelihood of having a Down's syndrome baby for a 40-year-old mother is one in 110, rising to one in 30 if the mother is aged 45 or over. It is important to note that the majority of babies with Down's syndrome are born to younger women, only because the overall birth-rate is higher in this age group.

The *Daily Telegraph*, on Friday, 21 June 1991 carried an interesting article on this subject, written by the Health Services correspondent, David Fletcher:

Risks 'Greater' in New Test for Down's Babies

A recently developed test used on pregnant women to detect Down's syndrome and other abnormalities in their babies, carries a considerably higher risk than the longer established amniocentesis test, a report on more than 3,200 women says today. It found that 14 per cent of women undergoing the new chorion villus sampling test lost their babies compared with 9 per cent of those tested by amniocentesis. Earlier this year, the chorion villus test was suspended at John Radcliffe Hospital, Oxford, after five in 320 babies whose mothers had undergone the test were born with severe facial and limb abnormalities. Dr Tom Meade, chairman of the Medical Research Council working-party which carried out the study, said chorion villus sampling carried a small extra risk but its advantage was that it could detect abnormalities earlier. He said: 'The study provides firm evidence to help pregnant women considering pre-natal diagnosis weigh up the small risk against the benefit of earlier diagnosis.'

The study, carried out in seven European countries, found there were significantly fewer surviving children in women tested by chorion villus sampling compared with amniocentesis. There were more spontaneous miscarriages and more foetal deaths in the mothers who underwent chorion villus sampling. A report of the findings, published in *The Lancet*, says: 'The results of this trial suggest that the policy of chorion villus sampling in the first trimester [first three months of pregnancy] reduces the changes of a successful pregnancy outcome by 4.6 per cent in comparison with second trimester amniocentesis.' Chorion villus sampling is used in about 50 hospitals on about 3,000 women a year, mainly in her late thirties and forties who have a statistically higher risk of having a Down's syndrome baby. The study says it is unable to confirm or refute any link with limb abnormalities in newborn babies. Chorion villus sampling involves analysing part of the placenta as early as eight weeks into pregnancy. Amniocentesis involves withdrawing a sample of fluid around the baby in the womb, but cannot normally be carried out until about 16 weeks into pregnancy. A league table of test-tube baby clinics to show which achieve the best results was urged by Dame Mary Donaldson, chairman of the Interim Licensing Authority, yesterday. She said the success rate of the 53 centres varied from nil to nearly 40 per cent, yet the public had no way of comparing their achievements.

Respiratory changes during pregnancy, a shortage of breath or an irritant cough, are not uncommon, but are unpleasant for the mother as well as for the baby. The herbal remedy Echinaforce can be taken safely for this condition, or Aconite 30C taken about four times a day is also a suitable homoeopathic remedy.

Another complication is premature birth, which is a birth that occurs before the thirty-seventh week of pregnancy, and this is often caused by placenta praevia, haemorrhage, high blood pressure, toxaemia, or respiratory conditions. Here the mother-to-be should immediately consult her doctor or mention it to her health visitor or midwife. Once again, the homoeopathic remedy Aconite 30C is suitable – three to four times daily – for a period of about seven days.

Long-term back trouble should be mentioned and if osteopathic or chiropractic treatment is required, the practitioner should always be informed of the pregnancy. Often back trouble is caused by pelvic problems which indicate a functional disturbance and this can easily be remedied, even by cranial osteopathy. This is often caused by a bilateral anterior sacrum maintaining an antalgic stance, or sometimes an increased lumbar lordosis, moving upwards and backwards by rotation. Such problems can result in hormonal imbalances, usually between the pineal, pituitary and thyroid glands, and the ovaries, which then govern the circulation in the sympathetic nervous system. It could cause other musculoskeletal disturbances with vertebral lesions which impinge on nerve roots and inhibit blood supply to the Fallopian tubes and the endometrium (the lining of the womb and the state of the cervix), which refers to the sympathetic and the sacral nerves. It is very important for women with long-term back problems to have this corrected. I have had several patients who miscarried because of back problems, so it makes sense to seek treatment for this condition before getting pregnant.

There is another complication I have come across a few times when a pregnant mother exposes herself to too much sun, or if she takes too many saunas. Women who take hot baths or saunas during early pregnancy can triple the risks of losing their baby. The risk of spina bifida or brain defects is also increased.

It is a known fact that in other mammals, exposing very young foetuses to heat can be dangerous, whether it be caused by fever in the mother, or external conditions. With very hot water or hot saunas, especially during the first six weeks of pregnancy, the risk increases two or threefold. In the USA a study of 22,762 women confirmed the increased risk of abnormalities in the foetus.

A healthy lifestyle is of course always important, but never more so than during pregnancy. It is widely thought that taking a sauna is part of a healthy regime, but in the case of pregnancy, common sense is called for. It is much more sensible to concentrate on a wholesome diet, stop drinking alcohol, stop smoking and stop taking any other forms of drugs. We can read how important this is in an article in *The Observer*, on Sunday, 24 May 1992, written by their science correspondent, Robin McKie, entitled *Heart Attacks Determined in the Womb*, from which I quote selectively:

> A group of scientists has found that heart conditions – as well as diabetes and reproductive disorders – appear to be triggered by events that occur before victims are born. Other ailments such as lung disorders and high blood pressure may arise in a similar way, and the work they are doing in trying to improve health by improving lifestyle is important, but not as important as the events that can occur before conception, in combination with forces that acted upon the foetus forming in the womb,

which will already have determined its susceptibility to certain diseases. Professor David Barker, Head of the Medical Research Council Environmental Epidemiology Unit at Southampton University, says that maternal malnutrition is the main problem, and that in the future Health Service officials may have to rethink completely their advice to adolescent girls who are preparing to become mothers. Professor Barker began his research 10 years ago, when he became dissatisfied with evidence that suggested diet and other factors were the causes of heart disease. In affluent areas of Britain, where people eat high cholesterol diets, rates of heart attacks and strokes remained low. Having expected the opposite, he began to look for other factors, and decided to examine those that might affect the developing foetus. A major boost for this work was the discovery of health records in Hertfordshire, Preston and Sheffield, which were compiled in response to official concern over the puny stature of working-class recruits from the Boer War. When researchers traced those babies who had been born underweight, and who had low weights a year after birth, they found that these infants had grown up into adults who tended to have heart attacks in middle life. They were also prone to diabetes and high blood pressure. The particular results showed failure to grow in infancy was followed by impaired glucose responses, poor blood-clotting and high cholesterol levels, while high blood pressure was a result of impaired growth in the womb. These growth failures were linked strongly with a mother's nutritional level. A woman who was in a poorly fed condition before she became pregnant, and could not properly feed herself while her baby was growing in her womb, was at significant risk of having children who had diabetes, heart attacks and other illnesses 40, 50 or 60 years later. For instance, if nutrition is lacking during the formation of the insulin-making cells of the pancreas, their functioning will be impaired and a person is likely to become diabetic decades later. Indeed, these problems can take even longer to take effect. During the Dutch Hunger Winter of 1944–45, when the Nazis attempted to starve the people of Holland, it was found that women who were pregnant at that time gave birth to babies of normal weight. However, the females who have since grown up are now tending to produce small babies. The development of their reproductive organs in the womb had been damaged during the Hunger Winter. Prof. Barker explains: 'The embryo is not like a clock that ticks at an absolutely fixed rate. It makes

115

trade-offs. If nutrition is restricted, it will divert what is available to those cells that are of the most importance, and away from cells that will not become important until much later in life. In other words, the embryo will trade off long life for survival. It is therefore crucial that a woman keep herself well nourished during pregnancy.'

I lost a baby cousin to meningitis, which is an inflammation of the brain lining and can be caused by germs, bacteria or a virus. If bacterial meningitis is diagnosed early and treated promptly, most cases will make a complete recovery. Currently there are about 3,000 reported cases of bacterial meningitis in the UK. When babies have a fever, are refusing feeds, are vomiting, are very dozy, show a pale and blotchy skin, are fretting, or display a rash, purple spots or bruises, contact your doctor immediately. Should it be diagnosed as meningitis, Aconite 30C can be safely given alongside the conventional treatment prescribed by the doctor, and if the baby is in distress and cannot bear to look at light, give it Bryonia 30C.

Yet another distressing complication is Rubella or German measles. This too can be very serious. Firstly, I would advise strongly that if you are planning a family, and if you have had measles, always take a homoeopathic potency of measles to make sure that any miasma (leftover from a former inflammation, virus or infection) in your body, is cleared. This highly infectious viral disease, which can be spread by coughs and sneezes, is definitely more serious in adults than in children and takes a high toll on one's immunity. If you have not had German measles, or are not sure, in order to minimise the risk of rubella during pregnancy, it would make sense to take a homoeopathic immunisation of Rubella 30C. Should you be in contact with a rubella case during pregnancy, consult your doctor, and take a rubella nosode 30C. In all conditions where German measles or measles have been or are involved, take 15 drops of Echinaforce three times a day. If a fever is involved, Aconite 30C is very helpful, and so is Belladonna 30C. Sulphur 6C should be taken for a rash and, in the case of a very high temperature, Bryonia 30C may be taken. However, all possible effort should be made to ensure that you avoid contact with rubella or German measles during pregnancy, for your sake and that of the unborn child's. Most children are immunised against measles, mumps and rubella with the MMR injection, but for parents who are principally opposed to immunisation it is important to consult a homoeopathic doctor who will advise you of other preventative measures that may be taken.

116

Yet another complication is the fairly common complaint of sore nipples. If the nipples are cracked use St John's Wort Oil together with Seven Herb Creme. If the nipples are sore because of mastitis or a breast abscess, Echinaforce should be taken or Megazyme to overcome the infection.

Between three and five days after the birth of the baby a new mother may be tearful or aggressive, and show signs of anxiety or sadness. It is estimated that 65–70 per cent of new mothers experience these feelings. The emotional change, which can be attributed to the changes in the hormone levels due to the baby's birth, are called 'baby blues' and usually do not last very long. In any event, a little Vitaforce and Ginsavita can help.

If, prior to pregnancy, the mother-to-be has had some allergy problems, these may rear their head after the birth and it is advisable to take a homoeopathic remedy such as Harpagophytum – ten drops three times daily – which helps to keep allergies under control. If it is a form of hay fever you would be well advised to take Pollinosan. Remember that there are many effective homoeopathic and herbal treatments for allergies. It is claimed that some 40 per cent of people in Britain have one or other form of allergy, and this is because generally the immune system is less effective than it used to be because of environmental or atmospherical conditions. Therefore, new mothers should take good care of themselves and make sure that they get enough rest. Old folklore used to advise: 'Nine months pregnant – nine months rest'. Studies certainly show that the body needs some twelve months to fully recover from the trauma of birth. It is very noticeable that during the period immediately after the baby is born the mother is more prone to illness than usual.

In the women's section of the *Glasgow Herald*, Friday, 29 November 1991, I read an article regarding the excellent care in hospitals for newborn babies. It said that for almost all British babies the first sight of the world into which they are born is a hospital maternity sheet. These days it is unlikely that an adult can point out to their offspring the house where they were born. Yet, there is something very beautiful about giving birth in your own home, and it certainly gives me great pleasure to drive past the house where I was born. Unfortunately, this is not the way the government wants it: hospital deliveries have been a consistent feature of the recent health policy in Britain and 99 per cent of births in Britain take place in a hospital. Delivery at home is very much frowned upon.

Maternity care in the Netherlands is very different, and so it surprises me that in Britain it is maintained that the birth of a new baby should be given as much care and attention as possible and should therefore take place in a medical centre, such as a hospital or maternity unit. If the present system allows maternity care in the community there is no good reason why mothers shouldn't be allowed a home delivery, which is already favoured by the majority of Dutch mothers.

Teams of doctors, midwives and health visitors in Britain can work very well, but I am sure that the individual and personal care of a home delivery is very much better for mother and baby bonding, especially as the baby is brought into the family from the moment it is born. Other children in the family feel very much more involved and young children in that family tend to have fewer problems with accepting the newcomer. In the case of a hospital delivery, the arrival of a new baby is often threatening to a young child as its mother disappears and reappears shortly afterwards with a helpless new baby, the centre of everyone's attention. Too often in such circumstances the toddler expects this new baby to usurp his or her place in the mother's affection.

The Royal College of Obstetricians advocates that it is better to have births taking place in hospitals or maternity clinics. When I look at the maternity care in the Netherlands or in other countries, I beg to differ. As most births are conducted by midwives anyway, I think that it would be wonderful if the mother could be delivered of her baby at home providing there is a good understanding between the midwife, health visitor and general practitioner. On the other hand, statistics do not lie and when the NHS started in 1948 with its maternity service, the number of fatalities at birth was 38.5 per thousand births, and today that is down to 8.3 per thousand. This greatly improved figure, however, still does not match Dutch statistics and so I sympathise with those women who would prefer a home delivery, providing good maternity care in the community was available. If a forceps delivery or a Caesarean section is required, this will, of course, always have to take place in a hospital.

It is quite frightening to learn that in Scotland one out of every six babies is delivered by Caesarean section; a trend in childbirth that has grown in recent years. I am rather worried about the increase in Caesarean sections as it appears to have become a routine method of delivery for babies who are at risk. A Caesarean section used to be seen as one way of reducing the risk of peri-natal mortality. Death in childbirth is rare, but a Caesarean section increases the risk appreciably. The *Glasgow Herald*, 22 July 1991, stated that the Senior Registrar at the Glasgow Queen Mother's Hospital believes that women underestimate the risks involved in a Caesarean section. He felt that they have become so common that many mothers fail to appreciate the extent of the surgery. It is a fairly extensive operation which involves the opening of the abdomen and the womb itself to deliver the baby. These days it appears to be down to the preference of obstetricians whether to deliver a baby in the natural way or by Caesarean section. I feel that Scotland is following in the footsteps of America, where up to 35 per cent of babies are born by Caesarean section, because American doctors are ever mindful of the possibility of litigation should the baby be handicapped. Sometimes Caesarean sections are performed to speed up the delivery, which I feel is completely wrong.

I have read that in the sixteenth century an impatient midwife would blow sneezing powder at the mother-to-be's nose if labour went on too long and even today there are some widely varying views on the subject. Different cultures clearly have different habits and thoughts on the matter. There is birth squatting; giving birth while seated in a bath tub; underwater births; and in Thailand one of the favoured ways is for the woman to lean back against her husband's body while he digs his toes into her thighs. Perhaps, as the article suggests, we should go back to the time-tested birth practices, instead of resorting to surgery. Remember that I have already mentioned some of the possible drawbacks of these kind of deliveries in the chapter on cranial osteopathy.

Another reason why doctors claim to prefer hospital deliveries is because of 'cot death', or Sudden Infant Death Syndrome (SIDS). There is no good reason for this because this usually affects babies between the age of one and five months. I remember how upset my family was when a very good friend phoned me in despair because her baby son had died, yet another victim of cot death. There is no satisfactory explanation for this occurrence, but such a traumatic event can leave the parents with great emotional scars. There are action groups in the USA who believe that it is caused by a nutritional deficiency, but this has not been proven. The position in which the baby sleeps may be important and it is now thought, as the result of research, that SIDS is more common among babies who sleep on their stomach. Therefore, babies that like to sleep on their stomachs should be encouraged to lie on their back or side, and in order to discourage them from rolling over onto their tummy in their sleep, you may like to consider using a safety harness. Temperature in the baby's room should be comfortable, but not too warm, with light blankets, and remember that sleeping in a smoke-free area is important, as indeed it is for adults.

The government has done little to encourage research into the incidence of SIDS. Various action or research groups have their own theories, for example, the chemical content of the urine has been analysed and an unusual composition has been found, and studies have been made of the magnetic forces around the location of the cot, and of geographic stress. Recent research has investigated the possible link between cot death and flame-retardant substances in the baby's mattress, but this has not yet been found to be conclusive.

In a report brought out after research in the Netherlands it was claimed that since mothers had been advised to sleep babies on their front, the incidence of cot deaths has trebled. Cot death has also been linked with social factors such as single motherhood, the young age of the parents, poverty, or bacterial influences. SIDS has been significantly defined as 'the sudden death of any infant or young child that is unexpected by history, and in which thorough post-mortem examination fails to demonstrate the adequate cause'.

The many reports I have read have brought me no nearer a satisfactory conclusion as to the cause of Sudden Infants Death Syndrome.

In an Australian paper in May 1980 I read about Collarenebri Hospital, where, after a very frustrating decade, the crib death-rate was cut to almost zero by the use of vitamin C. This story is related in the moving book by Dr Archie Kalokerinos, *Every Second Child*, where he maintains that the use of vitamin C was essential. I quote a passage from his newsletter, dated January 1983:

Buried in the *Bristol Mirror* of England, for Saturday, February 5 1820, was the following item: 'AWFUL OCCURRENCE – Thursday morning, a man, apparently enjoying the same state of health as usual, suddenly dropped down dead at the feet of his wife, who was at the time in labour. It is, however, pleasing to add that in the night of the same day, the woman was safely delivered of a fine boy, by Mr Earle, of Stoke's-croft, and the mother and child are likely to do well.' Now, more than one and a half centuries later, we know exactly why this young man dropped dead: it was a vitamin C deficiency. As was described by Dr Irwin Stone (Jour. Int. Acad. Prev. Med., 5:85–91, 1978), not only infants can fall victim to sudden death, but so can otherwise healthy adults who are depleting their vitamin C due to physical and/or mental stress. In fact, it is happening so much these days that it has been termed SADS, the A for Adult! Picture it: Bristol in February is cold and damp and this unfortunate fellow most likely skimped on his eating so that his pregnant wife was properly fed. She certainly got the fruits and vegetables, if there were any. He was worried, too, since by one contemporary authority, 32 per cent of newborns died in the first year. His wife's life, as well, back in 1820, was at great risk, and she was at that very moment in labour. His body and mind were under great stress that tragic Thursday morning. The meagre amount of vitamin C remaining in his body just wasn't enough to support the many metabolic processes depending on ample vitamin C, so his heart just stopped.

It is possible that there is a link to vitamin C supply, and expectant mothers should use vitamin C during their pregnancy. Another article on the same subject reads:

> We have further shown how an ascorbate deficiency may result in a sub-clinical scurvy which may escape detection at the time of immunisation. Parents may not get sufficient ascorbate in their daily diet and the mother may not be excreting ascorbate in her breast-milk. There may be a complete absence of ascorbate in infant formula-milk and in infant formula-food. The question is whether the recommended dietary allowance of 10mg of vitamin C is sufficient to provide fuel for the reticuloendothelial system to cope with this massive man-made immunological challenge.

I have seen small babies with tiny blisters on their lips and white patches on the tongue. Although this may look like thrush, it could also be an indication of vitamin C deficiency. If it is thrush, give the baby some Molkosan; a few drops in a spoonful of water will help to clear this quickly.

Sometimes complications can occur if the baby is under-fed, which are not always recognised early enough. Therefore, regular attendance at the post-natal clinic is essential. I must also stress that I am strongly opposed to the latest fashion for heating baby's milk or food in a microwave oven, and the same applies to the sterilisation of the baby's food utensils.

At the birth of one of my daughters, my wife went into labour a month early. All the signs were there, the doctor and midwife were in attendance, and dilation was advanced. Then everything stopped. If the baby is not ready to appear, leave it to nature. The next day a medical friend advised my wife to go for a brisk walk in the woods behind our house and, if the time was right, that her labour pains would surely start again. Well, my wife and I did go for that brisk walk, but the baby decided that it wasn't quite ready to arrive, and stayed in place for another month, just as our calculations had suggested. Fearing an infection because of my wife's earlier dilation, she was advised to take preventative measures. She took Echinaforce – fifteen drops three times a day – and all was well. When nature was ready the birth took place without any further complications. I often worry that this is not taken into account when induction is decided upon and when labour is started artificially. This should only take place if absolutely necessary because of the risk to both mother and baby. Castor oil with some strong coffee is a much more natural way. Midwives in previous generations used to advise an oil-bath or an enema. To my mind this is better than any artificial induction.

If it is necessary, however, the midwife or doctor will decide to make a small incision if the skin if stretched too tightly, rather than see the skin tear. These are minor adjustments to facilitate the birth process, and an incision will mend much quicker and better than if the skin is torn.

13

Infertility

Over the years I have seen many couples who have asked me for help because of infertility. I have often been upset when I have had to say that there was no hope. To my surprise, one of my nieces came to me with this problem and, having discussed the situation with her and her husband, I could not give them much hope. I suggested that they might like to make enquiries about a test-tube baby or about artificial insemination. With medical guidance they eventually decided to opt for the latter. We were delighted for them when, after a while, my niece told us that the treatment had been effective and that she was expecting twins. Indeed, when her time came she gave birth to a healthy set of twins, a son and a daughter. However, a year after the birth of the twins she came to tell me that she was pregnant again, without any medical interference or assistance, and in due course she gave birth to yet another baby.

My long-time housekeeper was also very concerned about her only daughter. She was concerned that she might never become a grandmother, because her daughter had still not managed to become pregnant, despite trying for a number of years. From what I was told I feared that the daughter might have endometriosis, and after vainly trying to help her, they were advised to try for a test-tube baby. The result was that she became pregnant with triplets. Of course, they knew about the increased risk of a multiple birth with this treatment, but still they were astounded, and initially slightly shocked. My housekeeper was delighted and became a grand-mother three times over all at once.

Because children are an outward sign of commitment in a relationship, having children is like the seal of approval. If the couple are very happy, children are the most precious things they can give each other and share together. This reminds me of a very amiable couple in their late thirties, who after many years of exhaustive tests, were told that there were no specific problems, and yet everything that had been tried had been unsuccessful. They had heard about a new treatment method and came to ask how I felt about GIFT – a method in which the eggs are removed, mixed with the husband's sperm and then replaced in the Fallopian tube. The success rate of this treatment is not too high, but in their case it worked on the third attempt and she became pregnant. Her pregnancy was not completely trouble-free, but a healthy baby daughter was born and they were extremely happy.

There are quite a number of methods available now for overcoming infertility, but considering the complexity of some of these methods, I always emphasise that any natural methods should be tried first. I have come across some wonderful surprises with patients of mine, and some children, who are now at our local secondary school, probably would never have been there, if the mother had not gone to such great lengths to conceive. One couple who had been trying for 17 years asked me for advice. She had some circulation problems, and I suggested that these be attended to first, before starting on a pregnancy programme. I prescribed the required remedies, and also suggested that she take a fairly high dose of vitamin E. Totally out of the blue – after nearly three months – she came back for her next appointment, agitated because she had missed a period and didn't know what to think of it. Had things been left too late and was this the onset of the menopause, or could she possibly be pregnant? Tests proved positive and she and her husband could not believe their luck. I was thrilled to see their reaction at the wonderful news, and their surprise and astonishment was complete when it was confirmed that she was expecting twins.

There has been so much publicity on the subject of infertility and we have all heard or read some incredible stories. A little while ago I came across another strange one in an American magazine: researchers had found that while tea had a negative effect on women's fertility, one caffeinated, short drink a day was enough to increase the chance of conception. Some of these unusual stories about fertility are not surprising given that the inability to conceive a child affects one in six to eight couples at some stage in their lives, and can cause profound distress. Normally couples have a 90 per cent chance of achieving conception within one year. If there is a longer delay they should seek advice.

Investigations into infertility problems take time. The main systems which need to be checked are those of ovulation, the proper production and passage of eggs from the ovary, spermatognesia (production of sperm), and also the mechanics by which the egg and sperm can meet to produce a fertilised egg, or zygote. It seems that if infertility problems originate in the male it is usually because of a low sperm-count. Oligospermia is a condition of insufficient male hormones or blocked sperm tubes for which there can be a number of reasons, and is symptomatic of insufficient sperm production.

Female infertility can be caused by a blockage or abscess in the Fallopian tubes. In the case of misalignments, I have found that osteopathic treatment can help to overcome certain problems and by manipulating and re-aligning the position of the womb I have been able to help patients to overcome some infertility problems.

One rare case comes to mind of a lady who had been trying for children for several years, and all the relevant medical tests had been performed but to no avail. Her husband's sperm-count was adequate and her ovulation was regular, and yet, she did not conceive. When I looked at her back I discovered an unusual deviation in her bone structure and I became suspicious that this could prevent the sperm reaching its goal. I contacted a friend of mine who specialised in gynaecology and asked him to give her a medical check and pay particular attention to her back. He confirmed my suspicions and she was taken into hospital for a minor abdominal operation, and since that time she has had five children.

Conventional first-time treatment in infertility cases involves inducing ovulation either by hormonal methods or by way of surgery, and, depending on the outcome, a decision can be made in favour of embryo transfer or IVF (In Vitro Fertilisation) which has been introduced as a treatment for women who have damaged, blocked or even absent Fallopian tubes. The GIFT method has progressed over the years. The development of ovarian follicles is assessed at regular intervals by ultra scanning, including blood and urine tests. Chorionic gonadotrophin is used which can allow the eggs to be recovered 36 hours later. The follicle fluid is usually sucked out using an instrument called a laparoscope or under ultrasound guidance. An average of six eggs can be transferred at this time, and the embryologist selects the best for transfer as the eggs have different potentials for fertilisation. With IVF treatment the eggs that are recovered are usually incubated in culture media for four to six hours to help them mature before insemination. A fertilisation rate of between 80 and 90 per cent is achieved if there is nothing wrong with the sperm. The embryologist judges whether everything is normal and of the right size and then the embryo is implanted in the womb by way of the cervix. The success rate is presently around 30–40 per cent.

These methods have also been adapted for egg donation, to be used in cases where women cannot produce eggs of their own. These are fairly expensive methods, but very worthwhile if the outcome is successful. Some couples have offered me considerable sums of money if only I could help them become parents. Money just cannot buy conception, it either works or it does not, but never underestimate nature, because a lot can be done to help it along. Recently, I met a beautiful and talented young ballet-dancer who told me that she would not have been here if it had not been for the help I gave her parents when they came to see me nearly 20 years ago to discuss their apparent infertility.

The advice I gave them was simple. Sometimes homoeopathic remedies can help rectify a low, male sperm-count and there are also natural remedies to help men reach full erection, such as ginseng, Ginkgo biloba, or Masculex. Some general tips for conception are:

1. Intercourse should take place every second day during the woman's fertile period
2. The woman's hips may be elevated with the aid of a pillow, so that the knees are bent during intercourse
3. The male sexual organ should remain in the vagina for a while after ejaculation has taken place
4. Refrain from using lubricants
5. Stay quietly in bed for at least half to one hour after intercourse has taken place. Do not take a hot bath or shower until well afterwards

It is always important that the menstrual cycle is regular, and if the problem is thought to be with the female partner, the first thing to be done is to regulate the periods. Some herbal remedies can be helpful here, such as Femtrol, together with the MST Formula. This provides a very good base for regulating menstrual periods. The programme can then be continued with the prescription of some additional vitamin E. I have found that Biovital is ideally suited under these circumstances. Biovital, sometimes referred to as the 'Master Formula', is a complex multiple vitamin and mineral supplement. Four tablets supply 100 per cent or more of the US recommended daily requirement of 10 important vitamins and minerals. These essential nutrients are included in a special foundation of glandular concentrates, herbal extracts, and other natural food factors, to provide complete nutritional support for all body systems.

The desired effect has been achieved, even in the case of endometriosis, by taking the remedy Ovarium, together with three 500 mg capsules of Evening Primrose Oil, taken last thing at night.

If there is no obvious reason for infertility, and the menstrual cycle is regular, I will sometimes try to bring the normal cycle of menstruation out of balance for a little while. I have used Ovarium and Sepia to de-regulate the normal cycle and sometimes found that as a result after a few months conception took place. These things depend so much on the individual, and once the practitioner has a good idea of the person's medical history and personal background, it is easier to be of help. For example, a 28-year-old woman came to me for advice. She had been married for just over two years and was upset because she had not yet been able to conceive. I found out that she had had several operations for the removal of fibroids and with the help of Petasan, a high supplement of vitamin C, and Steroplex-MF, her wish came true and to her great delight she conceived. The Steroplex-MF supplement, which is suitable for both men and women, provides a variety of nutrients that must be present for sexual gland functions.

If, after tests, I find that there are dietary deficiencies, I often advise the male partner to take a course of Zinc Plus. This remedy contains zinc picolinate and iodine. The body's stores of available zinc appear to be small and have a rapid turnover rate. Iodine, an essential micronutrient, plays a key role in proper thyroid function. If a man's sperm-count is really low, an improvement will be noticed if he takes Biovital and extra vitamin E and the already mentioned Zinc Plus remedy.

Sometimes I also suggest homoeopathic remedies such as Conium 30C, Agnus 30C, or Lycopodium. Unfortunately, a low sperm-count can be caused by the male having had mumps during puberty or adolescence. Excessive smoking, alcohol indulgence, use of steroids, or an accumulation of poisons or waste material in the system, can also result in a low sperm-count. In such circumstances I prescribe Petasan, which is a good cell-renewal remedy, in combination with a remedy called CPS (Cellular Protection System). CPS contains a high concentration of anti-oxidant nutrients in a base of unique herbal extracts and other natural compounds. Beta carotene, vitamin E, vitamin C, selenium, zinc, and manganese all have anti-oxidant functions. Riboflavin helps regenerate anti-oxidants after they have neutralised free radicals. The anti-oxidant complex also provides pycnogenols from grape seeds and green-tea extract. These substances are 50 to 200 times more potent than vitamin E. Curcumin, the yellow pigment of curcuma, and Nacetylcysteine, a stable form of the essential amino acid cysteine, are also powerful anti-oxidants. CPS supplies concentrated extracts of cabbage, garlic, ginger and Klamath blue-green algae. These foods contain a broad range of anti-oxidant nutrients, which make CPS the most comprehensive anti-oxidant formula available.

If you have a low sperm-count it is advisable to refrain from intercourse during the period building up to ovulation, in order to increase the chance of conception.

Whether I am asked to help with male or female infertility I always suggest that the patient revises his or her diet. Take care of your nutritional requirements with a good wholesome diet, wheat germ is particularly important. This nutrient has a high vitamin E content; 100 g of wheatgerm contains as much as 30 mg of pure vitamin E, and is therefore invaluable under the circumstances. Furthermore, the likelihood of a premature birth can often be reduced by taking wheatgerm.

In the past infertility was treated with high doses of yeast, but considering today's more common problems of Candida albicans I dare no longer make this recommendation. The herbal remedy Aesculus hippocastanum (an extract of the horse chestnut) may be taken – ten drops, three times day.

In some cases of infertility I have also used acupuncture and osteopathy as both these methods may succeed where others have failed. This just goes to show that there is a very wide variety of treatments which can be used without any side-effects. My final advice is that you should never give up hope. Remain positive and believe, when nature decides, your wish will come true and you will find yourself pregnant.

14

Endometriosis

Endometriosis is a mysterious condition where rogue cells from the lining of the womb – the endometrium – also grow in other parts of the body, frequently on the lining of the abdominal cavity and on the surface of the organs in the pelvic area, but also sometimes in the eyes, nose or lungs. These adhesions can have a normal activity, proliferating and bleeding in tune with the monthly cycle. It is estimated that 40 per cent of endometriosis sufferers are infertile. It has also been suggested that one in 10 women of child-bearing age could be suffering from this condition. The cause is still very much a mystery, but there are a number of theories, none of which has been proved conclusively. One theory claims that blood leaks out of the ends of the Fallopian tubes into the abdominal cavity because of an inefficient immune system. I have also read that it can be attributed to faulty tissue carried to other parts of the body by the lymph and the bloodstream. Yet, another theory maintains that the fault lies with the foetal development in the womb.

Quite often, there is a family history of endometriosis or it can be linked to a previously contracted disease. When first discovered in 1860 by Von Rokigansky it was regarded as an incurable gynaecological disease. There are many theories on this subject, such as the impartition theory, the embolic theory and the coelomic metaplasia. In short, endometriosis still baffles the medical profession. Why some women are affected and others are not is not known, because the origin of this condition has not been conclusively proven. Research done at the University of Chicago concluded that on average it may take as long as 10 years before a woman is diagnosed as suffering from this condition, because the symptoms are often dismissed or ignored.

Because of the suspected involvement of the immune system, it is important that this is given priority, and once again the initial requirement is a well-balanced diet. Although it is generally thought that women with endometriosis cannot bear children, this is not always the case. Diet plays a most important part in the treatment of endometriosis. I nearly always test women for any allergic reactions or tendencies, and I carefully check their diet for deficiencies of food-combining.

From the work by Dr G.E. Abraham and Dr C. Fredericks, it may be deduced that certain foods and matter containing oestrogens are likely to have an effect on this disease. As food patterns have changed so much and so many nutrient deficiencies have become apparent, causing an excess production of oestradiol, which is a self-proliferation factor, it is important that the diet be closely watched.

Dietary habits should also be checked with regard to vitamin, mineral and trace element contents. Before and around conception, a high content of B vitamins and essential minerals is desirable to maintain high levels of enzyme saturation. Ovulatory maturation and embryonic development involves the highest rate of cell replication in the human life-cycle and so requires a high local availability of inter-cellular energy. The conclusion by Schweppe for women suffering from endometriosis was that only permanent complete elimination of endocrine influences can cure endometriosis.

Also important is Riboflavin, or vitamin B2. This is essential for the adrenal gland to function and therefore controls stress reactions. Since women have a higher sensitivity to stress, they appear to be less fertile and since lutenising unruptured follicle – LUF – is associated with a higher trait anxiety, the suggestion is that stress about infertility in general induces subfertility in stress-prone women to the LUF syndrome. Riboflavin deficiency also causes hormonal imbalances and is essential for liver function, the clearance of steroids and normal hormonal functions.

Vitamin B6 is also absolutely essential because this vitamin, above all others, encourages the production of progesterone. Some research has indicated that women with endometriosis have an imbalanced oestrogen and progesterone production because of their monthly cycle. Women with endometriosis are often prone to depression and anxiety and a B6 supplement can give them a boost.

We often hear that women who suffer from this condition have a low energy-level and a magnesium deficiency may be the cause of this. Often there is a reduced dietary intake, absorption and utilisation of this mineral, symptomised by insomnia, cramps, and so on. The immune system in such women is less effective, and magnesium may have to be supplemented.

While on the subject of vitamin and mineral deficiencies I cannot omit the mention of zinc. I have seen wonderful results when this has been added to the diet, particularly with the thymus gland. The thymus gland has a strong influence on the T-cells and because endometriosis is an immune deficiency, a zinc supplement should also be seriously considered. As endometriosis is considered an auto-immune disorder, this would explain the symptoms of infertility.

Zinc and vitamin B6 are essential in order to produce adequate amounts of the sex-hormone, gonadotrophin, the release of which is necessary to stimulate the development of the ovum and therefore ovulation. While zinc is necessary for the metabolism, it is also very important for general health and fitness. A zinc deficiency can be the cause of an irregular menstruation pattern, irritability, depression and tiredness.

Another mineral that should be mentioned is selenium which has proved to be very valuable in the treatment of endometriosis. Selenium is also thought to have a strong influence on stiffness of the limbs. Evening Primrose Oil has also been useful for endometriosis. I remember that when I mentioned this supplement in relation with endometriosis on a radio programme, the response from listeners was overwhelming. Evening Primrose Oil has a general anti-inflammatory effect, probably due to its ability to increase the synthesis of PGE1 and thereby correct the level of prostaglandin. This substance is very important in any in-flammatory process and according to the Endometriosis Society it has been found to be of considerable relief if taken at the usual dosage – three 500 mg capsules when retiring for the night.

Endometriosis affects individuals in many different ways and when I see women with this condition, I can recognise the symptoms: a general lack of control over the body and acute mood swings. I can reassure them that they will feel very much better if they take Evening Primrose Oil. A healthy nutritional programme is also very important because it can correct deficiencies.

I have had a great many female patients who were desperate to become pregnant. In many cases they have had minor abdominal surgery, and the diagnosis of endometriosis has been confirmed. It is often so important that such a patient becomes pregnant, because that in itself may clear their condition. I must stress that there is no need to wait until the menopause when this condition will often disappear. The various remedies I have mentioned have often helped to overcome endometriosis at a much earlier stage.

One of my patients confided in me that she had tried to become pregnant for six years and admitted that she had accepted that because she had endometriosis it would be impossible for her to conceive. She was totally convinced of this fact and this is so sad, because a negative mind cannot possibly result in a positive outcome. We spoke and I persuaded her that, if she really wished to conceive, she should never give up hope. She said that she had had so many tests, internal scans, and seen so many doctors, that it had just made her thoroughly depressed. Both she and her husband had decided to forget about it. Her sadness and acceptance of the situation had caused her to gain excessive weight and we started to work on her depression and also on her body weight. Within three months she had lost most of her excess weight. Then I prescribed her a new homoeopathic and herbal remedy – Endobrit. She phoned me six weeks later to tell me that she had missed a period and she felt marvellous. I told her that it was early days yet, and that she should wait a little longer and then ask her doctor for a pregnancy test. The outcome was positive, she was pregnant and utterly delighted. During her pregnancy she was sensible and took no chances. The prospect of impending motherhood made her glow and changed her outlook on life and her personality. I used to look forward to seeing her in the clinic because she was so utterly happy. During her pregnancy, and even after the birth of her child, she emanated the radiance of a thoroughly fulfilled woman.

I am sure that Endobrit was instrumental in bringing about this change, but I also believe that things were helped by the initial change in her attitude. She had taken a positive approach and this so often is the secret of it all. I have seen women sitting across my desk who appear to have given up and resigned themselves to depression and failure. This will not help the situation and I find myself talking them into fighting back. They must never lose faith and hope that it is possible to overcome the barriers that have so far made conception impossible.

Endobrit, high supplements of vitamin C (as much as 2 g per day) together with Petasan (ten drops three times a day) and Ovarium, have successfully made fibroids disappear.

Another endometriosis patient, in her late twenties, had not been able to conceive in the two years she had been married and I prescribed some remedies to which she seemed to respond quite positively. Later, she told me that when she suspected that she might be pregnant she purchased a home-testing kit to see if her expectations were confirmed. These days most of these kits are bought in the hope that it will confirm a false alarm. This young woman, however, immediately phoned me to let me know that the home-testing kit had proved positive. It was a real tonic to hear her happiness and I had to calm her down and advise her to make an appointment with her doctor who would confirm her condition.

It is very rewarding to think of someone who has been so depressed, and to imagine her suspense on doing this test on her own at home, and then to see her delight at the positive result. I have seen a great many young women who have been troubled by endometriosis and who were doubtful about their ability to conceive. It is essential to encourage them and help them to remain positive, and in time many of them have been fortunate and have been able to conceive.

15

Exercises

One evening, coming home very late after a lecture, when everybody else was asleep, I peeped in to the baby's bedroom, hoping that the newborn baby would not be woken. What a picture of delight and perfection. The little one was totally relaxed and breathing steadily and I was reminded of the phrase: 'the breath of life'. The Hara breathing method – the breath of life – is what I was reminded of when I studied my very young daughter. It is important exactly where in our body our breathing takes place.

One of the exercises I have taught to young and old alike is an exercise I myself learned many years ago in China. One of my colleagues in the hospital there was tireless and capable of working very long hours, her endurance and appetite for work was phenomenal. Finally, I plucked up the courage to ask her what her secret was. She told me that she had been taught at a very early age the correct way to breathe and that this was what kept her going and gave her stamina.

The most critical time for everyone is at the time of day when they were born and that is the time of day when people tend to feel more tired than usual. I was born at 4 o'clock in the afternoon and I am very aware that my energy is at its lowest ebb at this time. This all changed when I was instructed in the Hara breathing method by this Chinese doctor. If I am given a few moments in between appointments at that time of the day, I lie down on the floor in my consulting room and practise Hara breathing.

Place the left hand on the stomach just fractionally below the navel and place the right hand on top. This creates a perfect balance in yin and yang. The flows of energy are improved by just this simple action. According to the Chinese, as the navel is the last connection that is severed at birth from the mother, this is the centre of the energy network. It is through the area around the navel that all energy intake occurs and this explains why the navel is sometimes called the 'abdominal brain'.

When studying acupuncture I learned that all the important reflex points for the heart, kidneys, liver, gallbladder, lungs, spleen, small intestine, colon and bladder, are all around the navel area, and that by stimulating or activating certain pressure points many problems relating to these organs can be relieved. The vegetative nervous system also lives around the navel and the more we are able to relax the better it will serve us. Therefore, by forming this small magnetic ring of balance with our hands it goes without saying that we will benefit.

Most children, from the age of four onwards, will move their breathing, some to the diaphragm, some to the chest; the latter is especially true of nervous or asthmatic people. But a baby with 'the breath of life' breathes correctly, from the lower abdominal area around the navel; the 'gate of all that happens', according to the Chinese.

I have taught many tense and anxious people how to breathe properly. With the left hand covered by the right hand, placed just below the navel, we breathe in through the nose and exhale through the mouth. We do this several times to get the feel of the rhythm. Then we imagine ourselves walking in nature, in a forest, along a beach, or in a beautiful flower-garden, where we can even smell the flowers, while breathing in naturally through the nose and deep down into the stomach. Exhaling takes place slowly through the mouth. This is the rhythm to keep: slowly in through the nose, deep down into the stomach, and slowly out through the mouth. It will not come naturally, but I can assure you that if you practise, you will notice the difference. A real feeling of well-being will come over you. Many people who I have instructed in this method in the past have let me know how pleased they are at having learned the Hara breathing method. There are many similar exercises, quite a number of which can be found in my book on stress-related and nervous disorders.

It is sensible for a mother-to-be to practise Hara breathing in preparation for the birth. From the moment she knows she is pregnant a woman will involuntarily be thinking about the birth of the baby and many will admit that they are not looking forward to the delivery because of the pain involved. They fail to grasp that pain is mostly brought on by fear. There is positive and negative fear, and, unfortunately, the fear of pain falls into the second category. Fear can be overcome by love and, as it says in the Bible: 'There is not fear in love.' Thinking of the love for a coming baby will be a great help. It is often said that God only helps those who help themselves, and therefore it is advisable that exercises are done to relax the muscles and the breathing.

Prof. Heinz from South Africa based his philosophy on the decompression method. He advocated a method where the mother was put in a sort of astronaut's costume so that air could be sucked away until there was no pressure on either the stomach or stomach wall. I think this is going a bit far, even though everyone agrees that everything within our power should be done to control pain. Pain can be successfully controlled by breathing or simple exercises for physical control, or with the help of a TENS machine. Often doctors prescribe tranquillisers to keep a patient calm and relaxed, but I am sure that most mothers-to-be neither need nor want that. Although the decompression jacket was reasonably successful, it was a cumbersome method and never became popular.

Another very helpful way for the expectant mother to keep her mind busy and focused is to use some acupressure points herself, and a great deal more about this can be found in my book *Body Energy*. There are acupuncture points which can be activated by gentle pressure to relieve labour pains and emotional pressure. All mothers-to-be nowadays are wisely encouraged to attend antenatal classes where relaxation and breathing methods are taught. Concentration exercises are also important. It was in antenatal classes that my wife was taught the Mensendieck technique, which she found to be excellent. She successfully used this method at the birth of all four children; although widely used on the mainland of Europe it is hardly known in Britain. Controlled breathing techniques are also helpful for people who have a tendency to hyperventilate.

Another useful breathing exercise is inhaling and exhaling through the mouth, slowly in and out, eight to 10 times per minute. Allow the effect to take place slowly. Keep the movement of the diaphragm to roughly 10 to 12 inhalations per minute, then gradually reduce breathing in and out to a frequency of six to eight times a minute. By doing this, the muscles become relaxed and the frequency can be increased and when one feels the need.

It is best to place several pillows under the head and also one or two pillows under the knees so that one feels comfortable when doing these exercises. Gentle leg movements are also a good idea during the exercise.

Always remember that a reasonable amount of exercise during pregnancy is safe, but it goes without saying that it should never be overdone. Recently, I had a pregnant patient who refused to take this advice and had insisted on continuing with her aerobics classes; inevitably she contracted a back injury. Unfortunately, it is much more difficult to put this right during pregnancy, because osteopathic treatment must be kept to the minimum. Always use your common sense, but never more so than during pregnancy when you should listen to what your body tells you and do no more than you feel comfortable with.

In the Netherlands, lots of women use their bicycle to get from A to B, whether pregnant or not. Many pregnant women continue cycling until the very last moment. Cycling is good exercise, as is swimming and walking. Most women who swim regularly have strong abdominal muscles which help them during birth. It is different with horse-riding, where one must take greater care than usual because a simple fall could be fatal. Tennis or badminton are also perfectly safe, as long as you feel comfortable. It would make sense, however, not to start any new types of sport during pregnancy; these can safely wait until after the delivery. Avoid jumping in any shape or form or any weird physical contortions, and be careful how you bend down: always bend from the knees and not the back. This advice is the same whether pregnant or not. Many women who have suffered back pains during pregnancy will instinctively take it a bit easier, and I should point out that long-term back pain can indicate kidney or bladder problems. If this is the case it is safe to use the herbal remedy called Cystoforce – ten drops three times daily.

It is also helpful for pregnant mothers, when they wake up in the morning, to walk about on tip-toe for a little while. This will help the back and stomach muscles. Remember to walk tall, wearing low-heeled shoes. Use a fairly firm mattress which will give you more support. To relieve leg or foot cramp, flex the foot while lying down, and if seated, keep the legs straight, and with both heels on the floor, pull the toes towards the knees. If standing, put all your weight on the affected leg and massage it.

Once the baby has arrived make sure that you have a comfortable chair to sit in when feeding your baby. Ensure that you are well supported and that feeding your baby is a pleasure and not something to be endured.

Some pelvic floor exercises will help keep back problems at bay. They are quite easily done: lie on the floor with legs bent and slightly apart and the arms folded. Breathe out while lifting or pushing the pelvis forward, then relax. Then, sitting on the floor, lean back until the stomach muscles tighten, hold this for as long as is comfortable, breathing normally, then breathe in and sit up straight again.

Lie flat on your back on the floor with the knees bent, feet slightly apart, resting your hands on your thighs; then lift your head and shoulders, and, stretching forward, breathe out slowly, and touch your knees. Don't worry if this cannot be done comfortably, but keep trying. Breathe in slowly and relax. Again remember the Hara exercise where you slowly breathe in, filling the stomach with air, and then slowly exhale. Do this about 10 times.

I saw an exercise in India many years ago which is very simple, but very useful. This exercise is called arti-arti, and to my knowledge is not practised in relaxation classes in Britain. Lie on the floor with arms spread wide and make yourself comfortable; you might like to use some cushions. Concentrate on relaxing the whole of the body, starting with the toes, feet, ankles, calves, knees, thighs and so on. Slowly move up along the whole of your body and concentrate on relaxing every limb. When you are fully relaxed, lift your hands from your wrists, upwards and downwards in rhythm with your breathing; at the same time, do the same with your feet, moving your toes up and down. So, as your hands go upwards, your toes also go upwards, and vice versa; breathe in and out in the same rhythm. This is a simple but very useful exercise for expectant mothers. *Getting into Shape* is a helpful guide to post-natal exercises, written by Gillian Fletcher, an obstetric physiotherapist with the National Childbirth Trust. Don't forget that exercise is equally important after childbirth.

Some lymph drainage is also very beneficial and can be achieved through massage, using a flowing technique; with both hands following each other, in such a way that they overlap. Start very lightly at the outset, gradually increasing the pressure as you go along the line of massage, always starting at the extremities and working towards the heart. This is very good for the lymph system. The lymphatic system's job is to nourish and cleanse the tissues of the body; this includes the breasts. There are about eight pints of blood in the body which carry nutrients to all the tissues and then remove carbon dioxide and various toxins. The lymphatic system has a great deal of work to do, and because of environmental pollution there is a lot of waste material to remove, so it is advisable to do everything possible to improve the lymph flow.

The lymph system mainly works during sleep. Therefore, it is important to make sure you get enough sleep. Do not sit up in front of the television until the early hours of the morning, thinking you are resting. During pregnancy, make sure that you get at least a minimum of seven or eight hours' sleep or bed rest.

Let me remind you that clothing should be light and loosely fitting and make sure that no straps or elastic cut into the flesh. Pregnant women often wear their bras too tight because of the increase in their bust size, but the digging of straps into the muscles and blood vessels can cause a considerable amount of discomfort.

Make sure you keep your exercises simple and do them regularly. Many mothers-to-be or new mothers are worried about stretch marks and losing their figure, so make time for these exercises and drink plenty of water as you lose some body fluid due to perspiration. Doing these exercises with enthusiasm can make your pregnancy an enjoyable time; a time of great anticipation for the big day when you will hold God's little gift lovingly in your arms.

Useful Addresses

Auckenkyle
Southwoods Road
Troon
Ayrshire KA10 7EL

Billings Ovulation Method
  Centre
58b Vauxhall Grove
London SW8 1TB

Billings Natural Family
  Planning Centre
196 Clyde Street
Glasgow G1 4JY

Bioforce UK Limited
Olympic Business Park
Dundonald
Ayrshire KA2 9BE

British Acupuncture
  Association
34 Alderney Street
London SW1V 4EU

Down's Syndrome Association
155 Mitcham Road
London SW17 9PG

Enzymatic Therapy
Hadley Wood Healthcare
67a Beech Hill
Hadley Wood
Barnet
Herts EN4 0JW

General Council and Register of
  Naturopaths
Frazer House
6 Netherhall Gardens
London NW3 5RR

General Council and Register of
  Osteopaths
56 London Street
Reading
Berks RG1 4SQ

Nature's Best
1 Lamberts Road
Tunbridge Wells
Kent TN2 3EQ

Bibliography

Thomas Bartram, *Nature's Plan for your Health*, Grace Publishers, Bournemouth

Harry Benjamin, *Everybody's Guide to Nature Cure*, Thorsons Publishers, Wellingborough

Dr Evelyn Billings and Ann Westmore, *The Billings Method*, Fowler Right Books, Leominster, Herefordshire

Phil Bosmans, *Leven de Moeite Waard*, Lannoo Publishings, Tiel, the Netherlands

Denis Brookes, *Cranial Osteopathy*, Thorsons Publishers, Wellingborough

Dr Andrew Lockie, *The Family Guide to Homoeopathy*, Penguin Books, London

Ronald R. McCatty, *Cranialsacral Osteopathy*, Ashgrove Press, Bath

Dr Carolyn De Marco, *Take Charge of your Body*, The Well Woman Press, Winlaw B.C., Canada

Lennart Nilsson, *A Child is Born*, Faber and Faber, London

Joseph Chilton Pearce, *Magical Child*, Bantam Books, Toronto, Sydney, London, New York

Diana Raab, *Getting Pregnant and Staying Pregnant*, Patterson Printing, Alameida CA94501, USA

Marion Stroud, *The Gift of a Child*, Lion Publishing, Tring, Herts.

Dr Thomas Verny with John Kelly, *The Secret Life of the Unborn Child*, Sphere Books, London

Dr A. Vogel, *The Nature Doctor*, A. Vogel Verlag, Teufen, Switzerland

Dr A. Vogel, *Anders Beter Worden*, UGN Publishing, Elburg, the Netherlands

Index